Prescribed Malnutrition

An Oncology Nutrition narrative review

Diana Artene

Copyright © 2024 Viorela-Diana Artene

All rights reserved.

The content of this book is exclusively the intellectual property of the author. Reproducing this book and any part of it in any manner without an explicit written permission from the author violates the copyright law.

First Edition: 1 September 2024

ISBN: 9798338004920

Fair warning to non-health care providers: I'm not sure if this book is for you as, at times, things can get quite technical. You may skip over the tougher parts, and if you'd like to shed light on the conflicting nutritional advice you've perhaps received over time, you're welcome to give it a try. Most people would like to sort the hype from the facts.

Disclaimer

The information presented in this book has a general educational purpose; it is not meant to replace professional oncology nutrition recommendations. The author does not accept responsibility for any adverse effects individuals may claim to experience, whether directly or indirectly, from the information contained in this book. Readers are solely responsible for their own healthcare- and nutrition-related decisions. Patient-appropriate oncology treatments and the appropriate supportive care need to be personalized.

"Consider how hard it is to change yourself, and you'll understand what little chance you have of trying to change others."

- Jacob M. Braude.

TABLE OF CONTENTS

INTRODUCTION TO ONCOLOGY NUTRITION 1

EXAMPLES FROM BREAST CANCER SETTINGS ... 11
Chapter 1 – Obesity 13
Chapter 2 – Sarcopenic obesity 23

BEHAVIORS THAT MAINTAIN MUSCLE MASS 39
Chapter 3 – Mediterranean diet 41
Chapter 4 – Physical activity 71

BEHAVIORS THAT AMPLIFY MUSCLE LOSS 87
Chapter 5 – Non-compliance 89
Chapter 6 – Alcohol intake 122
Chapter 7 – Smoking 132
Chapter 8 – Polypragmasia 148
Chapter 9 – Veganism 161
Chapter 10 – Alkaline diet 182
Chapter 11 – Intermittent fasting 196
Chapter 12 – Ketogenic diet 210

INSTEAD OF CONCLUSION 227
ABBREVIATIONS 231
REVIEWED SCIENTIFIC LITERATURE 232

INTRODUCTION TO ONCOLOGY NUTRITION

There are **two main** beliefs when it comes to oncology nutrition: "Cancer feeds on animal protein" and "Cancer feeds on sugar." And... maybe "You should take some supplements" too.

The "Cancer feeds on animal protein" belief is quite popular because a cancer diagnosis frequently comes with a juicer, with *The China Study* book, and with a welcome in the pseudo-oncology industry customers' community. However widespread, this belief ignores that proteins are digested in the human body. Thus, if you have this belief, it would help to acknowledge from the get-go if in the quest for the Holy Grail of cancer cure, you have given up on human anatomy.

Humans don't feed on proteins. We feed on food containing proteins, broken down during digestion into amino acids, so these can pass through the intestinal wall. Leaving aside the fact that there are many types of animal-based and plant-based proteins, we can biochemically call them "animal protein" or "plant protein" based on their content of essential amino acids. After their intestinal protein digestion, the only difference between "animal proteins" and "plant proteins" is that the plant ones don't provide all essential amino acids in the amounts required by humans' physiology. What we get from animal- or plant-based protein digestion are:

- All essential amino acids – after eating "animal protein."
- Only some essential amino acids – after eating one single food containing "plant protein."
- All essential amino acids – after eating more plant foods that contain complementary proteins.

If "animal protein" is carcinogenic, so would be combining "plant protein" food sources, which is recommended to vegans and vegetarians to get all the human-required essential amino acids. And keeping the emphasis on the garments while disregarding the bricks needed to repair the wall has no clinical benefit.

Professional oncology nutrition guidelines recommend a daily protein intake above 1g and, if possible, up to 1.5 g/kg of body weight during all stages of active oncology treatments (Muscaritoli M. e., 2021). Nevertheless, many people who advise oncology patients are not aware of oncology nutrition guidelines. Many disregard the overall quality of the patients' diets and their ability to chew, swallow, or tolerate otherwise generally healthy foods, ignore their ability to self-regulate their emotions without using eating as an antidepressant, and just focus on elaborate stuff like immunonutrition. Just that immunonutrition brings no benefit to well-nourished patients, as macronutrients are the foundation of human survival, not micronutrients (Klek, 2014).

What a patient diagnosed with cancer gets from avoiding "animal protein" during active oncology treatment is too few essential amino acids, which gradually amplifies the diagnosis-related and treatment-related catabolic state. This is even more detrimental during the surgical period because wound healing requires a higher protein intake (Weimann, 2021).

We can obtain optimal muscle anabolism and proper wound healing from a varied diet that combines animal-based and plant-based proteins. Still, animal-based foods should represent the majority of the protein intake (i.e., ≥65%), as translating popular cancer prevention recommendations to clinical oncology settings is insufficient to counteract the catabolic nature of the disease and its many treatments (Ford, 2022).

The "No sugar, no cancer" belief looks a bit more logical from a cancer biochemical point of view, as Otto Heinrich Warburg discovered that the type of malignant cells he studied in the 1920s were different from benign cells:

- having more glucose transporters and kind of acting like a glucose black hole,
- using glucose in the presence of oxygen as most benign cells would in hypoxic conditions, the energy-inefficient aerobic glycolysis being called ever since the Warburg effect (Warburg, 1956).

However, although all cancer cells can use aerobic glycolysis, all cancer cells don't have to. "Cancer" remains a generic word that covers many diseases, completely different from one another, even when we're talking about the same body localization. If there is one feature that different types of cancers have in common, it would be high metabolic adaptability. Still, many people prefer to keep it simple and extrapolate, ignoring the nuanced, personalized medicine. And more, much more ignore the nuanced, personalized oncology nutrition.

And also, it sounds kind of healthy. But the Warburg effect is about glucose, not about sugar. While consistent online dietary recommendations are lacking for patients during and after cancer treatment, even when it comes to the NCCN (Champ, 2013), there is no oncology diagnosis associated with the professional recommendation not to eat sugar.

Professional nutrition recommends limiting sugar to moderate intake. Moderation. No extremes.

And we only recommend moderation because:

- Even in the cancer cells that choose to use more glucose for whatever reason, this remains about glucose, not about sugar, and:
  - **Glucose can come from other carbohydrate-rich foods**—like fruits, beetroot, potatoes, bread, spaghetti, whole grain morning cereals, tomatoes, or avocado—the idea that cancer gets glucose only from sugar being non-sense.
  - **Glucose can be made inside the human body through gluconeogenesis**—a metabolic pathway that renders cancer cells even more aggressive when the glucose intake gets too low (Grasmann, 2019).
- Cancer cells can adapt to glucose deprivation and continue to proliferate by using fatty acids (Monaco, Fatty acid metabolism in breast cancer subtypes, 2017) and ketones (Martinez-Outschoorn, 2012).
- The intermittent pattern of access to pleasurable foods is the behavioral basis of eating addiction, the attempt to completely avoid one's preferred foods leading to overeating episodes, followed by even higher emotional need for avoidance, followed by even lower self-control (Fletcher, 2018).
- There is no benefit in increasing patients' distress as chronic stress itself may create a pro-metastatic environment (An, 2021).
- Patients' fear of cancer recurrence, body image dissatisfaction, uncertainty intolerance, and widespread internet use may lead to orthorexia, and orthorexia is not healthy eating (Waterman, 2022).

Cancer metabolism is far more complex than the popular but simplistic assumptions used to encourage patients to follow all sorts of dietary restrictions that would somehow starve cancer. While these many well-intended ideas feed patients' hope, the price for the short-term emotional relief is long-term increases distress and protein energy malnutrition.

Some cancer cells don't even bother using aerobic glycolysis, forcing it on the nearby stromal cells while maintaining absolutely normal metabolism. This boss-like ability to delegate hardship is called the Reverse Warburg effect, which has been demonstrated in luminal breast cancer cells (Pavlides, 2009). It is one of the features of more resistant breast cancers being correlated with lower survival (Witkiewicz, 2012). Nonetheless, we have a study performed on 740 real breast cancer surgery specimens showing that:

- only 40% of the metabolically analyzed tumor specimens used the Warburg effect,
- 7% used the Reverse Warburg effect,
- 9% used both,
- 44% used neither (Choi, Metabolic interaction between cancer cells and stromal cells according to breast cancer molecular subtype., 2013).

100 years later, we know today that the malignant cells that choose to use the Warburg effect can stop using it whenever necessary and just sit there dormant by switching back to the use of the Krebs cycle as a perfectly normal cell—metabolic pathway called the Crabtree effect (Smolková, 2010). Moreover, chemo and radiotherapy resistance is maintained through oxidative phosphorylation, not through aerobic glycolysis (Uslu, 2024).

Additionally, completely independent of any glucose intake, HER2+ breast cancers use fatty acids to resist treatment and metastasize to the brain (Ferraro, 2021).

Other types of aggressive cancers, among which high-grade ovarian serous cancer (Braicu, 2017), bladder cancer (Xiao, 2022), pancreatic cancer (Swierczynski, 2014), EGFR+ Non-Small-Cell Lung Cancers (Eltayeb, 2022), and BRAF+ melanomas (Turner, 2022) also default to using fatty acids to resist treatment and metastasize rather than utilizing the all-known aerobic glycolysis. Unlike the clear-cut assumptions that arose from preclinical studies performed on single-type cancer cell lines or on homogenous tumors developed in laboratory animals by scientists, a heterogeneous cancer developed by itself in a human had managed to do so precisely because it gradually developed so many genetic and metabolic adaptations that it can pretty much feed on whatever's available.

And the "whatever's available" includes even feeding on alive nearby cells—be they benign or malignant (Kroemer, 2014)—which are other aggressive metabolic pathways called entosis or cannibalism, found in more resistant cancer cells (Dziuba, 2023).

So, besides the old Warburg effect, different malignant tumors can use the Reverse Warburg and the Crabtree effects, gluconeogenesis, de novo lipogenesis, entosis, cannibalism, and the very Krebs cycle to resist treatment and metastasize. This practically means that even if the oncology patient ate nothing, cancer cells can thrive while the quality of life and the overall survival of the patient are lowered by malnutrition.

Oncology nutrition is not the current popular fad that butts heads with the ten others before it, sprinkled with blue scorpion venom and CBD drops. Oncology nutrition is first and foremost about accepting upfront that because of the high metabolic complexity, we cannot starve cancer. In any way.

Preventing and addressing malnutrition is the only role of oncology nutrition. There is no metabolic treatment for cancer. There is no anticarcinogenic food.

PRESCRIBED MALNUTRITION

Because of the complexity of the malignant metabolism, there are zero ways in which we can starve a malignant tumor grown in vivo on its own. And before the diagnosis, no food can prevent cancer as its etiology is highly multifactorial, preventing cancer by nutrition alone being another popular but inefficient make-believe.

Oncology nutrition is supportive care.

To be efficient, oncology nutrition practice requires one of the highest levels of professional nutrition training because the specialist must be able to personalize the dietary recommendations to the individual patient in front without perorating common generalities.

Professional oncology nutrition has nothing to do with the many common generalities. Increasing or limiting the intake of some macro- or micronutrients can, at times, be recommended based on both the disease(s) related features—cancer localization, immunohistochemistry, and treatment stage, and any other comorbidities—and on the patient's age, financial status, and level of emotional distress. It is important to avoid any excessive or insufficient intake that could contribute to treatment resistance by inducing malignant metabolic adaptations.

In cancer clinical settings, oncology dietitians can help the patient:

- by preventing the muscle loss associated with most treatments,
- by addressing the digestive side effects of the systemic ones,
- and sometimes, by also addressing the patient's need to use food for emotional comfort.

Oncology dietitians are rare though, many big hospitals hardly having one or two general dietitians, if at all. And this book is going to sound disrespectful to healthcare providers who don't play the self-proclaimed "nutritionist" game and just try to help patients with the general and popular advice they came across by reading a book or attending some conference lectures. But because of the Dunning-Kruger effect[1] most of us fell prey from time to time, the higher the expertise in the other professions, the more confusing the impact of the many advice that contradict each other to such an extent that most patients pretty much don't know what to eat anymore during treatment.

Nowadays, there are so many unprofessional diplomas available that it rains with "nutritionists." Also, there are many healthcare providers who think we're simply pointless and just replace our entire profession by printing the same copy/paste old ideas on all patients' discharge sheets as long as they're diagnosed with "cancer." Thus, in real clinical practice, what most patients get instead of personalized oncology nutrition recommendations specific to their own individual trajectory throughout the cancer treatment is non-personalized, unprofessional advice that became popular by sheer repetition. And that's about it.

But does it help a cachectic patient with pancreatic adenocarcinoma to receive the same xeroxed sheet as an obese patient with a low ER, HER2 negative breast cancer? Who does it help to say the same thing to a patient with a nasopharyngeal tumor undergoing chemoradiotherapy as to one with an EFGR-/ALK-/ROS1- triple-negative but PD-L1 positive non-small cell lung cancer undergoing chemoimmunotherapy? Or to one with an EGFR+ lung cancer taking Osimertinib? Doesn't it change anything nutritionally if a patient receiving internal

---

[1] The Dunning–Kruger effect is a cognitive bias in which a person's lack of knowledge in a certain area causes them to overestimate their own competence.

mammary lymph node radiotherapy also has a Helicobacter Pylori infection? Does anyone care if a patient recommended Tamoxifen could have other therapeutic and nutritional recommendations if she also has factor V Leiden mutations? Do we even ask? Is the patient under FOLFIRINOX treatment metabolically influenced similarly to the patient under bicalutamide treatment? And what if, alongside bicalutamide, he also has added docetaxel because his disease progressed to the bladder and now has hematuria—should we still change nothing about the copy/paste "cancer diet" recommended in some clinical settings on autopilot? Is it still business as usual if the patient receives chemoradiotherapy with cisplatin or with capecitabine? And do we say the same ol' same ol' to a patient with triple-negative breast cancer receiving adjuvant capecitabine alone? Would we just copy/paste the same text to all patients, even if some of the patients have uremia, severe anemia, secondary hemochromatosis, or 43 ml/min/1,73m2 eGFR?

Shouldn't we count these in when making professional dietary recommendations in oncology settings?

Can the system wipe away all these nuances that impact treatment efficacy and toxicity simply because "that's how it's been done since forever"?

If you are a healthcare provider and there are no oncology dietitians at hand, and the system requires that you also somehow address nutrition, it would be fair to at least write on the discharge sheet that the copy/paste text is non-personalized advice.

Nevertheless, sometimes, even when we don't have to say anything about things outside our area of expertise, we feel the inner emotional need to somehow help the patient, at least with some advice.

Any unprofessional advice is based on two primary factors:

- **The level of expertise one has in a specific area** – the higher the authority, the higher the drive to extrapolate it to areas where one has truly no professional training.
- **The level of emotional connection one has with the patient** – the closer the affected person, the higher the need to do something to help.

For the tumor, higher aggressivity means higher metabolic adaptability. For humans, higher tumor aggressivity means higher distress. And what gets out of the higher distress when doubled down by low expertise are simplistic clichés and nutrition extremes—prescribed malnutrition.

EXAMPLES FROM BREAST CANCER SETTINGS

Chapter 1

Obesity

Epidemiology dug for breast cancer roots in hair dye (Xu, 2021), antiperspirants (Allam, 2016), night shift work (Jones, 2019), street noise exposure (Sørensen M. e., 2014), environmental pollutants (Rodgers K. M., 2017), and in watching TV (Schmid D. a., 2014). There are many hypotheses, but to date, the only scientifically proven nutrition-related risk factors for breast cancer remain obesity and alcohol intake.

It is generally considered that increased body mass index (BMI) is associated with higher postmenopausal and lower premenopausal breast cancer risk. However, central obesity increases breast cancer risk independent of menopausal status (Houghton, 2021) or BMI (Chen H. e., 2023). And the coexistence of obesity and cancer family history may further exacerbate breast cancer risk (Cao J. e., 2024).

The good news is that obesity is a reversible risk factor, as we have old data (Eliassen A. H., 2006) and new data (Teras, 2020) showing that overweight and obese women who manage to lose 10 kg and keep them off obtain a decreased breast cancer risk as compared with those who do nothing about it.

The tricky news is that this weight loss must be fat loss to reap the rewards. Avoiding weight loss through starvation diets is important because these associate muscle loss—aggravating the increased weight gain tendency by increasing the fat deposited inside the muscles (Ahmed S. e., 2018). Attaining a normal body weight without improving body composition does not improve health and does not prevent breast cancer (Park Y.-M. M., 2017); normal-weight women by BMI but with excessive adiposity continue to have a higher breast cancer risk (Iyengar, 2019).

The bad news is that obesity is thriving worldwide, becoming more and more accepted as a normal part of one's identity that most people simply choose to do nothing about. We even have data suggesting that we're kind of doomed from birth, the baby girls born with high birth weight presumably having a higher postmenopausal breast cancer risk (Stephenson Babatunde Ojeifo, 2018).

So, we're all fat, we're all going to die anyway, the heck with obesity!

Nevertheless, both obesity and breast cancer remain issues worldwide.

Breast cancer patients who are obese at diagnosis have increased all-cause- and breast cancer-specific mortality risks (Chan, 2014), data showing that obesity is associated with worse breast cancer prognosis independent of stage (Robinson, 2014), immunohistochemistry (Harborg, 2021), and age (Copson, 2015).

The worse prognosis may be caused by the fact that baseline obesity is not only a risk and a prognostic factor for getting breast cancer but also a predictive one after you get it: some oncology treatments have lower efficacy and more side effects in obese patients, while others the exact opposite.

Breast cancer surgical treatments are technically more challenging in obese patients.

- **Therapeutic breast cancer surgery**
    o Obesity is an independent risk factor for infections across all breast cancer surgeries (De Blacam, 2012).
    o Obesity is an independent risk factor for venous thromboembolism events following mastectomy (Tran B. H., 2013).
    o Obese breast cancer patients undergoing mastectomy have a higher incidence of flap necrosis, independent of other comorbidities and tumor-specific characteristics (Wang M. J., 2021).
    o Obesity is correlated with more hematoma, reoperation, and nipple-areola complex loss following simultaneous therapeutic and contralateral prophylactic nipple-sparing mastectomies (Sonagli, 2021).
- **Reconstructive surgery**
    o Obesity is an independent risk factor for wound complications after mastectomy, with or without immediate reconstruction (Nickel, 2022).
    o Obesity is an independent risk factor for complications after breast reconstruction (Mrad, 2022).
    o Obese patients with breast reconstruction following mastectomy are more likely to experience surgical and medical complications having a higher risk of reoperation and wound dehiscence (Panayi, 2018).
    o Each unit increase in BMI correlates to 13% increased odds of implant-based reconstruction failure (Vaccari, 2023)
    o Obese patients have a 2-fold higher overall complication and device explantation rates for subpectoral implant placement (Asaad, 2023).
    o Obesity is a risk factor for complications following autologous breast reconstruction (Frid, 2024), and

even more so in the rare situations when obesity and malnutrition co-occur (Chiang, 2023).
- **Axilla surgical management**
    o The diagnostic performance of axillary ultrasound (Macaione, 2020) and MRI (Chen S.-T. e., 2022) for the preoperative lymph node assessment may be lower in overweight and obese patients.
    o Being overweight or obese at the time of surgery increases the risk of breast cancer secondary lymphedema (DiSipio, 2013), and postoperative weight gain further increases the risk (Shen, 2023).
    o Obesity is correlated with an increased risk of chronic pain after breast cancer surgery (Leysen, 2017).

However, some breast cancer surgical treatments seem to be less influenced by obesity:

- There is moderate evidence to support a higher risk for seroma formation in patients with heavier body weight, but this can be biased by the more extensive surgery (Kuroi, 2006).
- Goldilocks mastectomy is a surgical breast cancer treatment that can be offered to patients who are poor candidates for traditional methods of breast reconstruction due to obesity or other comorbidities (Richardson, 2012).
- Medical complications are higher in obese patients undergoing tissue expander and pedicled TRAM reconstructions, but no significant difference is observed in patients with latissimus and free-flap reconstructions (Hanwright, 2013).
- Partial flap loss, total flap loss, and complications in nonbreast reconstructions are not significantly different in obese vs. non-obese patients (Shin, 2016).

- Obesity is not associated with inferior locoregional control after breast conservation, which is a surgical treatment option regardless of the patient's BMI (Patel V. e., 2020).
- While caution should be exercised when performing oncoplastic surgery for breast cancer in patients with class 2 or 3 obesity (BMI ≥ 35 kg/m2), oncoplastic surgery is a safe procedure for these patients too (De La Cruz Ku, 2023).
- Autologous breast reconstruction has a lower surgical complication rate when compared to implant-based reconstruction for obese patients (ElAbd, 2022).
- Reconstructive surgeons should expect more postoperative complications and revisional surgery when performing autologous breast reconstruction in patients with recent massive weight loss (Sinik L. e., 2022).
- When compared to subpectoral reconstruction, prepectoral implant-based reconstruction is associated with a significantly decreased risk for complications, infections, and device explantation in obese patients (Asaad, 2023).

It is true that some systemic treatments have lower efficacy and higher toxicity in obese breast cancer patients.

- **Chemotherapy:**
    o Obese patients with early breast cancer have lower overall survival when treated with docetaxel-containing chemotherapy (Desmedt, 2020).
    o Obese breast cancer patients are less likely to achieve pathologic complete response = pCR (Wang H. e., 2021).
    o Obesity is associated with early recurrence after achieving pCR (Acevedo, 2022).

- o Obesity is associated with more neuropathy (Greenlee, 2017) and fatigue (Inglis, 2020).
- **Anti-HER2 treatments:**
  - o Overweight and obese patients with HER2-positive breast cancers are less likely to achieve pCR after neoadjuvant targeted therapy (Chen L. e., 2023).
  - o PCR rates are lower in overweight or obese patients with triple-positive primary breast cancers after neoadjuvant chemotherapy and anti-HER2 therapies (Di Cosimo, 2020).
  - o Overweight and obesity are risk factors for cardiotoxicity from anthracyclines, sequential anthracyclines, and Trastuzumab (Guenancia, 2016).
  - o Obese patients with HER2-positive breast cancers have a higher incidence of grade 3 and 4 adverse effects and more frequent treatment discontinuations (Martel, 2021).
  - o Obesity is correlated with worse overall survival in patients with metastatic HER2+ breast cancers who received Pertuzumab and/or T-DM1 (Krasniqi, 2020).
- **Anti-estrogenic treatment:**
  - o Obese patients treated with either Letrozole or Tamoxifen had slightly poorer overall survival than patients with normal BMI (Ewertz, 2012).
  - o Overweight and obese premenopausal breast cancer patients treated with Tamoxifen have lower overall survival (Sendur, 2016).
  - o The risk of venous thromboembolism with Tamoxifen looks higher in obese patients (Walker A. J., 2016).
  - o Aromatase inhibitors seem less effective in obese postmenopausal patients with HR+ breast cancers, but the size of the effect cannot be assessed (Ioannides, 2014).

- o Overweight and obese patients with early-stage breast cancers treated with aromatase inhibitors experience more arthralgia than non-obese patients (Beckwée, 2017).
- o Obesity is correlated with an increased risk of resistance to antiestrogenic treatment (Barone, 2022).

But the impact of obesity on chemotherapy remains unclear, while other systemic breast cancer treatments seem to either not be affected or work even better in obese patients:

- Obesity is correlated with better overall survival following immunotherapy (Woodall, 2020).
- Higher BMI is associated with better overall survival in patients with advanced HER2+ breast cancers (Modi, 2021).
- Overweight and obese patients with HR+ breast cancer have better responses to CDK 4/6 inhibitors (Yücel, 2024).
- Normal/low BMI patients with early breast cancer patients experience more severe neutropenia than patients with higher BMI during chemotherapy (Abraham, 2015).
- Overweight and obese patients with breast cancers are less likely to achieve pCR with body surface area neoadjuvant chemotherapy, but this might not be the case with actual body weight-based neoadjuvant chemotherapy (Wang H. e., 2024).
- Adding Abemaciclib to Fulvestrant or aromatase inhibitors prolongs the survival of patients regardless of BMI (Franzoi, 2021).

- There is no difference in treatment efficacy between normal, overweight, and obese women with metastatic HR+ breast cancers treated with Fulvestrant (Zewenghiel, 2018).
- Patients treated with Alpelisib and Fulvestrant show no difference in response according to BMI (Ge X. e., 2022).

Radiotherapy side effects are higher in overweight and obese patients:

- BMI ≥25 may be a risk factor for cardiac toxicity after radiotherapy for left-sided breast cancer, possibly because of the more frequent setup errors (Evans, 2006).
- BMI ≥ 25 is a significant predictor of acute radiation dermatitis (Xie, Risk factors related to acute radiation dermatitis in breast cancer patients after radiotherapy: a systematic review and meta-analysis., 2021).
- High BMI is predictive of a higher incidence of edema and pain during breast cancer adjuvant radiotherapy (Behroozian, 2021).

Except that the allotted negative impact of obesity on radiotherapy may happen in all women with bigger breast size, irrespective of BMI:

- Large-breasted women are more likely to suffer changes in breast size and shape after whole breast radiotherapy is delivered using 3D dosimetry (Goldsmith, 2011).
- Breast edema risk increases with more irradiated breast tissue (Verbelen, 2014).
- The larger volume of the breasts per se is the risk factor for the higher rate of acute adverse events and suboptimal final cosmetic outcomes in adjuvant breast cancer radiotherapy (Ratosa, 2018).

- There is a contradiction between preclinical and clinical findings, as although preclinical data underlines that adiposity could promote tumor growth and radioresistance (Sabol, 2020), clinical studies fail to show an increase in local recurrence in patients receiving adipose fat transfer after breast cancer surgery (Waked, 2017), and we even have clinical data showing that the prophylactic lipo filling before radiotherapy reduces breast tissue radio damage, improving reconstructive surgery outcomes (Gentilucci, 2020).

The issue is not only with baseline obesity but also with weight change after diagnosis. In 2002, the Journal of Clinical Oncology published a systematic review of 158 studies and underlined at the time that weight gain after diagnosis correlates with increased recurrence and mortality risk (Chlebowski, 2002). Further data points toward a higher impact for a post-diagnosis weight gain of more than 10% (Playdon, 2015). And although many patients with breast cancer gain some weight after diagnosis, those who gain larger amounts risk higher all-cause mortality, breast cancer-specific mortality, and recurrence (Pang, 2022). But before recommending weight loss on autopilot to overweight or obese patients, there is one more thing we should keep in mind: weight change doesn't mean only weight gain.

- **Weight change during chemotherapy** in patients with high-risk early breast cancers is associated with worse overall survival (Mutschler, 2018).
- **Weight loss ≥5% at 2 years** worsens the prognosis for patients with HER2+ early breast cancers, being correlated with worse overall survival (Martel, 2021).
- **Weight maintenance for up to 5 years** after diagnosis is associated with better survival, while a weight loss of >10% increases breast cancer-specific mortality (Jung A. Y., 2021). Moreover, a BMI loss exceeding 10% from

baseline to post-adjuvant chemotherapy predicts significantly worse overall survival (Chen H. e., 2023).

There is a J-shaped association between baseline BMI, the risks of recurrence, and overall survival. Baseline obesity is a risk factor for getting a breast cancer diagnosis and a negative prognosis factor since obese women frequently have more advanced stages of cancer at diagnosis. Nonetheless, the predictive impact is treatment-dependent: negative for some, neutral for others, and apparently positive for others. Thus, individualized risk factor evaluation, personalized recommendations, and shared decision-making are the keys to obtaining the best outcome for each individual patient.

Chapter 2

Sarcopenic obesity

One of the ways humans are treated like standard objects is the total body weight relative to height ratio, called Body Mass Index (BMI). According to the standard World Health Organization (WHO) definition, overweight refers to a BMI of 25 to 29.9 kg/m^2, and obesity to a BMI > 30 kg/m^2—with grade I from 30.0–34.9, grade II from 35.0–39.9, and grade III ≥ 40. By this index, 1 in 8 people was obese in 2022, as worldwide adult obesity has more than doubled since 1990.[2]

BMI formula was created in the 1830s by Lambert Adolphe Jacques Quetelet, a Belgian mathematician trying to define the "normal human" with no calculators, CT, DEXA, BIA scales, or any of the modern devices of our time—which is why he probably chose the simplest math. And after all these years, many still use it today to define normality.

It is true that BMI has no costs.

---

[2] https://www.who.int/news-room/fact-sheets/detail/obesity-and-overweight

It's quick and easy to calculate; thus, it seems like a useful tool that anyone can use regardless of low financial resources or time constraints. The sad truth remains that in many clinics and hospitals, there is no oncology dietitian. Or even a general dietitian, for that matter. Sometimes, the nurses try to cover the lack of professional nutritional services available to patients; other times, physicians try to address nutrition a bit in the little time they have for each consultation on top of their many other responsibilities. Still, obesity thrives worldwide in breast cancer settings regardless of good intentions, available resources, gastronomy, or culture.

Breast cancer-associated obesity is the elephant in the room most have no resources to effectively address, some having a bias against heavier patients, others shaming them for being greedy or for having low self-control, ignoring that weight loss might be as hard for patients as it can be for any of us. And although most have no awareness that breast cancer treatments cause weight gain by generating muscle loss, because baseline obesity and weight gain after diagnosis are correlated with increased mortality, in breast cancer settings, "Lose weight!" has become like a clinical mantra.

BMI is a heuristic, freely available, easy-to-use shortcut.

And as with any shortcut, it can lead to trouble.

Many assume that a higher number equals higher adiposity. But this is not a fact, as at the same BMI:

- Elite athletes can be misclassified as overweight or obese (Sundgot-Borgen, 2012).
- Older people have more adiposity than younger ones (Javed, 2022).
- Women have more adiposity than men (Romero-Corral, 2008).

- Postmenopausal women have more adiposity than premenopausal women (Opoku, 2023).
- Asians have more fat than Caucasians (Tan, 2004).
- Even South Asians Living in America have greater intermuscular fat and less lean mass, in addition to higher visceral fat when compared with Chinese Americans (Shah, 2016).

Differences also exist between Caucasians and Afro-Americans, Hispanics, Polynesians, Ethiopians, and Indonesians. Although scholars have requested gender-specific, age-specific, and ethnicity-specific BMI cut-offs for decades, the WHO has ignored these in the name of convenience (Deurenberg, 1998).

If we add in the fact that many busy clinicians do not weigh or measure the height of individual patients, just asking about these, then the epidemiological correlations made with BMI are frequently built on self-reported data (Freigang, 2020). And if you're a healthcare provider, just out of curiosity, what's stopping you right now from evaluating body composition in your clinical practice? Meaning? Access to proper measuring devices? Time to do it on top of all other things you have to do?

We are not standard objects as we can have different body shapes and sizes at the same total body weight and height. And letting aside that the BMI accuracy in predicting adiposity can be biased by age, gender, menopausal status, sedentariness level, and ethnicity, the correlations it makes population-wise bring no clinical utility to individual patients. In the era of precise medicine, using BMI to define a behavioral disease as complex as obesity in a therapeutic context as complex as oncology seems like a sunk-cost fallacy that ignores the actual human's metabolic or behavioral health.

Abdominal fat affects organs like the kidneys, liver, and heart more severely than the fat around the bottom. Women with normal BMI with higher visceral fat have a higher pre- and postmenopausal breast cancer risk (Houghton, 2021). After the diagnosis, normal BMI patients with higher visceral adiposity have worse overall survival (Dalal, 2014), more liver steatosis (Draisci, 2019), insulin resistance (Iwase, 2020), and cardiovascular toxicity independent of pre-existing risk factors and administered cancer treatments (Feliciano E. M., 2019). These increased risks among normal-weight healthy women and patients with breast cancers and greater visceral adiposity would go undetected by BMI alone.

Waist circumference measurement is a tool as simple, fast, and free to use as BMI, but a more accurate one that can be used as a proxy for visceral fat in the clinical settings where other body composition measurement options are not available (Felício de Souza Mamede, 2024). Nonetheless, many keep going with the flow of the abundantly published BMI epidemiological data, ignoring its lack of value in improving anything over the years.

Are we against admitting the lack of BMI efficacy?

Has it all gone down to publishing things to get published?

BMI says nothing about muscle mass, which is highly important both for maintaining metabolism to avoid weight change after diagnosis (Heymsfield, 2022) and to obtain optimal prognosis—in breast cancer settings, sarcopenia predicting higher toxicity (Rossi, 2019) and mortality (Zhang X.-M. e., 2020).

Sarcopenia can be quantitative or qualitative, being defined by low muscle strength plus either low muscle quantity or low muscle quality. Healthy skeletal muscle mass is vital for movement, thermogenesis, and metabolic homeostasis. It plays a central role in protein metabolism by serving as an amino acid deposit used to maintain protein synthesis in the absence of amino acid absorption from the gut and by providing hepatic gluconeogenic precursors in the case of too low protein intake or energy deficit (Wolfe, 2006). Although the muscle amount is not enough to define it (Sanchez-Rodriguez, 2020), in many published clinical trials, strength is not evaluated in any way, with sarcopenia being defined only as a skeletal muscle index < 39 cm2/m2 calculated using a software program by normalizing the cross-sectional area of the skeletal muscle mass at the L3 vertebra level based on computed tomography (Couderc, 2023). Most clinicians don't define sarcopenia in any way, ignoring for decades the skeleton in the hospital closet (Butterworth Jr, 1974). While most patients kind of perceive it as lowered strength and maybe fatigue. The majority miss it in obese patients diagnosed with breast cancers although myosteatosis and sarcopenic obesity are more prevalent than the low-quantity type of sarcopenia in these settings, the general concept of low-quantity sarcopenia being just more generally acknowledged.

Myosteatosis is low-quality sarcopenia, defined as the inter- or intramuscular infiltration of fat. It is an independent all-cause mortality risk factor, even in asymptomatic healthy adults (Nachit, 2023). Patients with myosteatosis and gynecological, renal, pancreatic, hepatocellular, gastroesophageal, and colorectal cancers or lymphomas have 75% higher mortality as compared to non-myosteatosis patients (Aleixo G. F., 2020). In breast cancer settings, there is less data about its impact than in other cancer settings because it is not acknowledged or measured on a day-to-day basis. Most healthcare providers working with patients with breast cancer have no awareness of the muscle quality impact on their work efficacy. In the few available studies, myosteatosis seems more present in patients with baseline obesity, and it is associated with a worsened prognosis (Sheean, 2021). However, the number of patients within these studies is low; thus, further research is needed to individuate myosteatosis' independent impact on prognosis in patients with different breast cancers. So, in addition to the total quantity of muscle loss popularly known as sarcopenia, myosteatosis may affect people with a normal quantity of muscle mass, be they normal BMI, overweight, or obese (Weinberg, 2018). And in the day-to-day clinical practice, muscle quantity or quality depletion after a breast cancer diagnosis may happen even in patients who do not reach the BMI cut-off for overweight or obesity.

Sarcopenic obesity is defined based on both skeletal muscle index and BMI, but even in this case, there is no consensus among scholars, while most clinicians have no clue of the body composition muddy waters. Researchers label a patient sarcopenic obese when they meet the criteria for both sarcopenia and obesity, and different international societies adopt different takes on this issue. In clinical practice, obese patients are seen as simply obese—being defined based on visual perception, with complete disregard for the quantity or the quality of their muscle mass. However, breast surgeons may need to ask about extreme dietary attitudes self-imposed after the cancer diagnosis and evaluate muscle mass in morbidly obese patients more carefully before surgery, as protein deficiency and sarcopenic obesity synergistically increase the risk of surgical complications independent of their surgical expertise (Dietch, 2015).

All proposed academic definitions of sarcopenia and sarcopenic obesity include the measurement of muscle mass, but there is no international consensus (Amini, 2019). The evaluation of fat deposition in muscles is even more complex, as it is accurately obtained only through muscle biopsy and only estimated by other means.

CT is considered the gold standard for myosteatosis evaluation, although an updated systematic review and meta-analysis of the available data found 32 different cut-off values (Ahn, 2021).

But while the academic best technique for measuring body composition seems somehow in the eyes of the beholder, the clinical best technique is the one that you've got, as cost, availability, and ease of use determine which option is better in clinical trials vs. clinical settings.

In clinical trials, besides BMI, waist circumference, waist-to-hip or waist-to-height ratios, and CT, there are other options that can also be used to measure body composition:

- There is some data on the use of ultrasound to assess muscle mass in older people, but future research is required to confirm this in both the sick and healthy populations (Nijholt, 2017).
- In younger patients with breast cancers, it is hypothesized that the pectoralis muscle area depletion on the MRI performed preoperatively after neoadjuvant chemotherapy could be a proxy for sarcopenia (Rossi, 2023).
- Dual-energy X-ray absorptiometry (DXA) is considered the next best thing (Buckinx, 2018), whereas:
    - no more than two body scans per year are currently advised for safety reasons;
    - in real-world oncology practice, many patients under endocrine therapy are not even prescribed one annual DXA for bone health evaluation (Amar, 2024).

Outside clinical trials, CT, US, MRI, or DXA are ignored for body composition assessment (Mortellaro, 2024). In clinical settings, bioelectrical impedance analysis (BIA) has been used to assess body composition since the 1960s as it provides a simple, portative, and less expensive alternative to radiology measurements (Thomasset, 1962).

However, the BIA devices using a 50 kHz single-frequency device with tetrapolar wrist-ankle electrode placement are the most widely used, and compared to DXA, they overestimate fat-free mass in patients with breast cancer (Bell, 2020). Many types of BIA devices accurate for oncology clinical practice have been developed over the years (Branco, 2023), with prices varying from 20 to 20.000 euros according to improved body composition accuracy—data underlining that measurements from one device to another are not interchangeable (Ward, 2019).

Although CT, US, MRI, and DXA are body composition measurement options for clinical trials, and while each budget-friendly BIA scale can be used in clinical settings to complete the BMI, none are used in most hospitals, as many clinicians default to self-reported weight and height data. Even though the preoperative BIA body composition measurement is useful in predicting the risk of complications following cancer surgery (Matthews L. e., 2021), many surgeons ignore it altogether based on the confusing studies that put the measurements made with BIA scales with single-frequency, 8 frequency, 16 frequency, and 32 frequency, with two, four, or eight electrodes devices, all as the same "BIA data," pretty much like labeling a tractor and a Lamborghini as an automobile.

If you are a healthcare provider, what body composition measurement could be the easiest to implement in your current clinical practice, from CT, US, MRI, DXA, BIA scale, and waist circumference measurements? And if you are a patient, has your body composition been evaluated in any way at diagnosis and throughout the many treatments?

It is important to know that many oncological treatments generate muscle mass loss, increased adiposity, and myosteatosis, even in patients who maintain the same BMI throughout treatments.

While older age is also associated with these conditions, they may occur at any age and across all cancer stages (Feliciano E. e., 2017). And although outside clinical trials, lots ignore sarcopenia and sarcopenic obesity altogether because they don't measure body composition and therefore don't visibly see them, these are factors that may influence therapeutic outcomes independent of personal expertise.

For instance, while it is generally considered that baseline sarcopenia is rare in non-metastatic breast cancer and that it does not predispose to surgical complications (Broyles, 2020), newer data shows that:

- Sarcopenia increases the risk of skin flap necrosis in patients with total mastectomy (Yabe, 2021).
- Preoperative sarcopenia correlates with an increased risk of severe complications in patients undergoing free-flap breast reconstruction (Jain N. S., 2023).
- Preoperative sarcopenia (Kim S. e., 2022) and sarcopenic obesity (Sadok, 2022) are associated with an increased risk of complications in women undergoing DIEP breast reconstruction (deep inferior epigastric perforator flap).
- The incidence of delayed wound healing, seroma, and bleeding is higher after expander breast reconstruction in patients with sarcopenic obesity (Nakamura, 2020).
- These risks increase after neoadjuvant chemotherapy, but the lack of international consensus for sarcopenia, myosteatosis, and sarcopenic obesity may result in bias (Lewis, 2024).

The consensus is that neoadjuvant chemotherapy is not associated with increased complication rates after immediate breast reconstruction, either with autologous tissue or implants (Sabitovic, 2023).

However, body composition is a predictive factor for breast cancer chemotherapy toxicity (Roberto, 2024):

- Baseline sarcopenia is associated with lower pCR rates (Aleixo G. F., 2023).
- Chemotherapy-generated sarcopenia increases the risk of severe postoperative complications such as surgical incision infection, respiratory failure, and postoperative hemorrhage, especially in the elderly (Su, 2024).
- Sarcopenia is a significant risk factor for neoadjuvant chemotherapy severe toxicity (Ueno, 2020), the 30-day morbidity after breast cancer surgery with immediate breast reconstructive surgery being higher in sarcopenic patients that develop more anemia throughout neoadjuvant chemotherapy (Jang, 2023). The administered substances may play a role, too. Patients receiving the docetaxel, carboplatin, trastuzumab, and pertuzumab TCHP regimen have a significantly higher risk of developing sarcopenia than those who received the anthracyclines and cyclophosphamide followed by a taxane AC-T regimen (Jang, 2022).
- Patients with non-metastatic breast cancer and skeletal muscle depletion (Huh, 2020), sarcopenia (Chen S. e., 2021), myosteatosis, or high visceral fat have significantly higher breast cancer-specific and all-cause mortality (Jeon, 2021).
- A higher increase in visceral adipose tissue is associated with shorter disease-free survival (Trestini, 2023).
- Among women with early-stage HR+ breast cancers, sarcopenia is associated with toxicity-related early treatment discontinuation (Saraf, 2024).
- Myosteatosis is associated with adverse events during chemotherapy for early breast cancer (Aleixo G. F., 2020).

- Sarcopenic patients with metastatic breast cancer have more grade 3–5 toxicity, shorter time to progression, and shorter overall survival (Aleixo G. F., 2019).
- Sarcopenia may be a risk factor for lower survival in patients with brain metastasis from breast cancer (Sim, 2024).

Furthermore, a normal BMI says nothing about being behaviorally healthy.

Humans' ability to stop eating is influenced by adiposity because the fat tissue is an endocrine one. Paradoxically, people with higher adiposity have higher satiety hormone (leptin) and lower hunger hormone (ghrelin), this being manifested as a lower ability to feel satiety and by feeling more intense cravings throughout the day—which is called leptin resistance (Barateiro, 2017). Regardless of BMI, excess adiposity generates the need to eat more, further increasing adiposity in a snowball effect amplified by crash diets that produce fast weight loss at the expense of lowered self-control (Kharbanda, 2022). Normal-weight women by BMI but with excessive adiposity don't become healthier, as losing weight without losing fat does not improve metabolic or behavioral health or oncology outcomes. That is why defining obesity by a number negates its' complexity and kind of separates patients into the good, the bad, and the ugly, without any clinical utility for preventing or for solving it.

Currently, there is no evidence that weight loss after a breast cancer diagnosis improves survival. Because of adiposity's impact on eating self-control and muscle's impact on metabolic maintenance, to improve prognosis, it is important to improve body composition by normalizing adiposity without losing muscle.

Just telling a patient not to overeat is not even close enough.

That is because although some patients might overeat to cope with distress, most don't. Without professional psychological support, patients who do emotionally eat usually continue to do so regardless of being told to stop, and even more so during the harsh systemic treatments frequently associated with high emotional distress.

This happens in reality exactly as in the case of healthcare providers who usually smoke more when stressed before getting themselves sick, who continue to do so after an oncology diagnosis due to the increased distress, irrespective of professionally knowing better. Patients are humans, too, and to prevent weight change after diagnosis, we must consider the disease, the treatment, and the human nature.

It may be well-intended to tell the patient to "Just lose weight!". But the reason why many patients don't just do it is that they are people, not robots equipped with tumors. A cancer diagnosis does not default to an improved lifestyle but to more extreme behaviors used to cope with the increased distress. And the fact that eating is the most used behavior to obtain relief from distress makes emotional eating and chronic dieting the other sides of a cancer diagnosis.

In breast cancer settings, we've known for years that many patients gain weight after diagnosis, mainly during chemotherapy, with no overeating whatsoever (Demark-Wahnefried, 2001). The main cause of chemotherapy weight gain is the treatment deregulated muscle protein synthesis/protein breakdown rate.

To maintain metabolism and avoid weight gain, this rate must be kept as even as possible throughout treatments:

- **Muscle protein synthesis** is the anabolic process that describes the incorporation of amino acids into skeletal muscle proteins. This is maintained by proper protein intake (Prado, 2020) plus regular physical activity (Li X. e., 2023). Thus, it takes both exercise and proper, individualized nutrition to have a healthy body composition or to regain it by reducing adiposity while preserving muscle mass (Kudiarasu, 2023).
- **Muscle protein breakdown** is the catabolic process describing muscle protein degradation into their amino acid precursors. This is amplified by chemotherapy, premenopausal women experiencing the most muscle loss and subsequent adiposity increase (Godinho-Mota, 2021). And, regardless of age, this gets even more amplified in polypharmacy (Prokopidis, 2023).

The early implementation of resistance training or combined aerobic exercises plus a proper nutrition intervention can keep the muscle protein synthesis/protein breakdown rate steady, which is especially important during neoadjuvant chemotherapy (Jang, 2023). However, systemic treatment toxicity is often somewhat implied and ignored in oncology, some healthcare providers and some patients alike doing nothing about intentional metabolic maintenance during chemotherapy.

And yes, it hast to be intentional.

Maintaining metabolism during chemotherapy cannot be achieved passively. To protect muscle mass and avoid sarcopenia's detrimental impact in oncology, the most basic oncology nutrition recommendation is not to lose weight. The most basic oncology nutrition recommendation is that patients diagnosed with cancer require a higher protein intake than the general population (Arends, 2017).

This gets higher in patients with baseline obesity as the anabolic sensitivity of postprandial muscle protein synthesis to the ingestion of a protein-dense food is reduced in overweight and obese young adults (Beals, 2016). This is even more important in elderly patients, as they are also more resistant to anabolic stimuli (Breen, 2011). However, data shows that healthy elderly with primary, age-related sarcopenia consume significantly less protein than their peers with no sarcopenia (Coelho-Junior, 2022). Why on Earth would anyone amplify this age-related sarcopenia-inducing tendency during sarcopenia-inducing oncology treatments by discouraging patients from eating meat?

Some healthcare providers think they can replace oncology nutrition by asking patients not to gain weight during the systemic treatment and to avoid red meat. But the red meat working definition contradicts even the color of meat in reality (Seman, 2018). The focus on BMI ignores the fact that weight loss doesn't equal fat loss, and that weight maintenance does not mean body composition maintenance. Then, there are two more things that kind of transform the NIKE motto "Just do it!" into frustrated rolled eyes instead of changed behavior: the patient's ability to digest foods during chemotherapy and the patient's socioeconomic status.

First, chemotherapy lowers patients' digestive capacity through mucositis, dysbiosis, and local inflammation (Walker J. e., 2023). Thus, many emotionally stable patients who understand and do their best to apply what they're told to do during chemotherapy find themselves unable to follow the recommendations, requiring dietary updates adequate to the lowered intestinal tolerability.

Neoadjuvant chemotherapy significantly affects body composition, as visceral fat may increase parallel with muscle depletion even when BMI remains unchanged (Iwase, 2016). Nonetheless, most healthcare providers have no oncology nutrition training, and both primary and secondary sarcopenia remain under-diagnosed and overlooked.

Moreover, the chemotherapy-generated sarcopenia can be obscured by the parallel increased adiposity if the clinical assessment focuses on BMI alone. And, for patients who start neoadjuvant chemotherapy with baseline sarcopenia, the risk of muscle mass loss during treatment is quite higher. Thus, to reduce the masking of muscle mass loss by the increased adiposity during chemotherapy and their detrimental consequences, body composition evaluation needs to be implemented in clinical practice as sarcopenia increases toxicity, decreases efficacy, and is worsened by chemotherapy (Jang, 2022).

Second, solving sarcopenia or sarcopenic obesity without counting in poverty has a fat chance (Eskandari, 2022). Maybe because of food insecurity, maybe because of main access to cheap but ultra-processed foods, these are more prevalent in poor countries and in poor areas of rich countries (Templin, 2019). Their detrimental health impact may be biased by lower educational level, higher sedentariness, chronic diseases, depression, and faster cognitive decline, as compared to people who have the time, finances, and knowledge to manage their eating behavior throughout their lifespan. And these socioeconomic factors become even more obesogenic in low-resource breast cancer settings (Sella, 2022).

We need to empower these women to stabilize their eating behavior where they are and with what they have, not to advertise weight loss for the sake of weight loss. The essential condition needed to have short-term chemotherapy side effects is that patients must be approached in a multidisciplinary manner, not only by the medical oncologists but also by the specifically oncology-trained physical therapists, psychotherapists, and dietitians:

- The medical oncologist evaluates the need for supportive medication.
- The oncology-trained physical therapist adapts the physical exercise plan to the general state of the patient diagnosed with a specific cancer during a specific oncology treatment.
- The oncology-trained psychotherapist evaluates and helps the patient counteract the emotional distress potentially generated both by diagnosis and by the many treatments.
- The oncology-trained dietitian evaluates if the patient's eating behavior is adequate to counteract these side effects and if she hasn't adopted extreme nutritional attitudes that may amplify their incidence and intensity.

Preventing weight change during chemotherapy and optimized body composition is possible with professional oncology nutrition, physical activity, and psychosocial support (Thomson, 2017). Still, many patients don't get these types of supportive care. Thus, when the treating physicians are overloaded with work, and the physical therapist, the psychotherapist, and the oncology dietitian are missing from the multidisciplinary team that should offer supportive care during chemotherapy, all these are usually passed down to the nurse's working agenda—who, besides her own responsibilities, must now also address the potential kinetic, nutritional and psychological side effects of the treatment with the basic information available that should theoretically replace three other professions she doesn't have.

Consequently, due to the muscular, emotional, and digestive side effects of chemotherapy, in the clinical settings where these types of professional, supportive care are not available—and even more so in patients with lower socioeconomic resources—what we get from neoadjuvant chemotherapy is upfront amplified sarcopenic obesity.

BEHAVIORS THAT MAINTAIN MUSCLE MASS

Chapter 3

Mediterranean diet

In 2010, UNESCO recognized the Mediterranean Diet as part of the Intangible Cultural Heritage of Humanity, as we can barely find it in the old rural parts of Mediterranean countries today. The traditional eating habits of people around the Mediterranean Sea used to provide a long, happy life, being abundant in vegetables, legumes, fruits, bread and other forms of cereals, potatoes, nuts, seeds, and kernels, olive oil, wine, and sweets, alongside different amounts of dairy, fish, poultry, meat, and eggs, according to the different geographical areas of each of these many countries.

As opposed to these old traditional Mediterranean ways, the "Mediterranean" diets sprung from the eating patterns observed in some villages in Greece and Italy in the late 1950s by Ancel Keys and then morphed into a restrictive diet built on the Seven Countries Study, the most applauded epidemiological study of the last century, and the practical basis of the low-fat diets promoted in the US ever since (Keys A. , 1980).

His hypothesis that saturated fat found in meat and dairy was the culprit for cardiovascular disease because it increases blood cholesterol preceded the Seven Country Study.

He first started to explore it in 281 American executives aged 45 to 55 who were followed prospectively by annual examinations since the winter of 1947-1948. Over the next 15 years, 32 of these directors developed coronary heart disease, all having high total cholesterol (Keys A. e., 1963).

Keys' hypothesis seemed to be in agreement with the Framingham Heart Study initiated in 1948 to investigate the American post-war cardiovascular disease epidemic. However, high cholesterol here was only one among the potential risk factors, alongside obesity, high blood pressure, and smoking (Dawber, 1966); for instance, it was known already at the time that smoking during stress increases cholesterol independent of any eating (Kershbaum, 1963). This was confirmed by the findings of the Western Collaborative Group Study (Rosenman, 1970) and by the Belgian Heart Disease Prevention Project (Kornitzer, 1981), which showed that the more competitive, stress-driven, type A personality is an independent risk factor for coronary heart disease.

Other scientists at the time disapproved that saturated fats were the cardiovascular disease culprit (Blackburn, 1975). Choosing to finger-point cholesterol in stressed middle-aged American executive smokers during the harsh financial struggles after the Second World War, as compared to relaxed elderly Greek village people while disregarding the other cardiovascular risk factors, looked kind of cherry-picked. Debates about the lack of external validity of Keys' studies were high, but they were and have continued to be ignored since the '80s US dietary guidelines (Astrup A. e., 2021).

Today, the scientific evidence against the saturated fat-cholesterol hypothesis stacks up day after day. Meanwhile, America has become fatter than ever and has more cardiovascular disease (Teicholz, 2023).

Like going to someone's house and choosing to see only what you're looking for while ignoring all else, so is the difference between the traditional Mediterranean ways and the subjectively designed diets called "Mediterranean". For instance, the first "Mediterranean" diet observational study performed on elderly people living in three Greek villages evaluated only eight types of foods: vegetables, legumes, fruits, nuts, grains, meats, dairy, and alcohol (Trichopoulou A. e., 1995). Even fish was not on the table until years later (Trichopoulou A. C., 2005). And these studies were not performed considering type A personality under stress or smoking, nor high blood pressure, sedentariness, or family history of cardiovascular disease.

The main problem with observational studies is that they can be so easily biased that whatever one would like to prove or disapprove, with statistics and semantics, can be. Only a few of the observational studies are adjusted for imprecise measurements or potential confounders. The many working definitions used by different authors contradict each other on the same topic. And while some authors state in the text of the article that their findings were likely to be affected by such details, they don't also write this in the abstract, which is the only part of the article read by most.

For instance, the freshly published Italian ORDET Cohort study concludes: "The adherence to a typical Italian Mediterranean diet protects against breast cancer development, especially among postmenopausal women, possibly through modulation of chronic low-grade inflammation" (Quartiroli, 2024). The study compares the effect of adherence to the subjectively defined Italian Mediterranean Index (based on an adapted version of the Greek Mediterranean Diet score), the Greek Mediterranean Index (based on the Mediterranean Diet scale), the DASH, and the EAT-Lancet scores. Besides, the Italian Mediterranean Index is shown to be protective only in postmenopausal women. In this study, no other

"Mediterranean" diet but the Italian was associated with decreased breast cancer risk. Not even the Greek one.

If, within the dark times, we remember how Albus Dumbledore advised Harry to turn up the lights and actually read the entire article, we might get a little more clarity on why this was the case:

- **Initially, there was no nutritional data or measured inflammation markers.** The original cohort of the ORDET study consisted of 10786 healthy women aged 35–69, residents of Varese Province in northern Italy, recruited between 1987 and 1992. At recruitment, information on lifestyle, menstrual and reproductive history was collected; height, weight, waist, and hip circumferences were measured; and blood and urine samples were given. However, the ORDET study design changed twice since its making.
- **The first change happened 2 and a half years into the study** when the diet was put on the table once the remaining 9144 women completed a semiquantitative food frequency questionnaire, self-reporting dietary habits over the preceding year.
- **The second change happened 22 and a half years into the study** when inflammatory markers measurements were performed in 2017. To add some oregano to the saga, these were not even evaluated within the ORDET study but copy-pasted from two other case-control studies. Moreover, the added data was each obtained with different kits; thus, ORDET statisticians standardized them and just reported the calculated results. Table 2 shows that the Italian Mediterranean Index was calculated for 214 postmenopausal women: 85 in the lowest and 29 in the highest tertile of adherence.

What is the relevance of the nonspecific C-reactive protein inflammatory marker patchworked within the study, which was statistically significant only in 29 out of 9144 participants of a study?

Mixing case-control with cohort data is common in epidemiology, though they're quite different.

Most studies backing up the "Mediterranean" diets are retrospective case-control ones that cannot establish causality and that are scientifically meant to be used for rare diseases. There are also prospective cohort studies that would be more appropriate for the not-so-rare diseases like the cardiovascular ones, cancer, or obesity, but while these can ascertain risks, they are more expensive to perform, take longer, and are harder to conduct. In the many available systematic reviews, although cohort studies directly contradict the hypothesis raised by the case-control ones, the difference is tossed under the rug, while the confusion is further amplified by availability bias:

- case-control studies are cheaper and easier to perform, thus more prevalent,
- but although they are more prone to selection bias and recall bias, because of the much higher availability, they have more weight in establishing general opinions for those who perceive case-control and cohort studies as the same tomayto, tomahto "data."

Availability bias is a heuristic used to make fast decisions based on popular rather than accurate information, which is frequently less acknowledged by the vast majority. Not only are case-control studies more readily available, thus more persuasive despite the higher bias and no power for causality, but their results can also vary from one to another based on the different indexes used to define the "Mediterranean" diet in each individual study: the Mediterranean diet score, the

Mediterranean diet scale (Willett, 1995), the Mediterranean food pattern (Martínez-González M. A., 2002), the Mediterranean Style Dietary Pattern Score (Rumawas, 2009), the Mediterranean Dietary Pattern adherence index (Sanchez-Villegas, 2006), the relative Mediterranean diet (Buckland G. e., 2009), and the Mediterranean Adequacy Index (Alberti, 2009) being just a few among the many invented.

No Italian Nona was asked in the '60s if she agreed with Ancel Keys' idea to replace butter with margarine or if she considered Grana Padano a non-Mediterranean food.

These different indexes are made-up questionnaires meant to summarize the self-reported adherence to a subjectively defined index by means of a calculated score. Some researchers consider them useful in evaluating eating trends that are deemed sufficient to develop public health guidelines. However, other researchers have underlined for decades that a more precise definition of the Mediterranean diet is needed if we strive for the accuracy and efficacy and that typical Mediterranean foods should be on the table (Bach, 2006). Nevertheless, there are at least 22 definitions of the "Mediterranean" diet (Hernandez Ruiz, 2015).

The lack of standardized guidelines is a limitation of the Preferred Reporting Items for Systematic Reviews and Meta-Analyses (PRISMA), reviewers making waters even more muddy by using suboptimal methods to assess risk of bias that give different results and thus are not interchangeable (van Enst, 2014), whereas the study design, sampling, follow-up, and confounding are frequently overlooked (Chrystoja, 2021).

Consequently, 60% of the available expert reviews do not apply appropriate statistics and do not comply with methodologic quality standards (Huedo-Medina, 2016).

The differences between what was consumed traditionally in the Mediterranean area and the many modern "Mediterranean" diets are even more striking among the interventional studies. For instance, another freshly published study performed in breast cancer settings—the Diana-5 study—shows that a "Mediterranean" diet doesn't help breast cancer patients prevent recurrence (Berrino, 2024).

According to the authors, the dietary intervention was based on Mediterranean diet principles, including some fermented food from the Macrobiotic tradition (miso, soy sauce, tempeh, umeboshi). The upfront intervention goals were to reduce:

- overall caloric intake,
- high glycemic index food: refined flour, potatoes, white rice, cornflakes,
- high insulinemic foods: sugar and milk,
- sources of saturated fats: red and processed meat, milk, and dairy products,
- trans fatty acids: margarines and industrial snacks and pastries, and
- protein intake, mainly animal proteins.

Just that their made-up macrobiotic, low glycemic index, vegetarian "Mediterranean" diet custom-designed for breast cancer patients completely ignored that:

- The idea that low-GI diets are superior to high-GI diets for weight loss or obesity prevention is an unproven hypothesis (Gaesser, 2021).
- There are no professional oncology nutrition settings recommending lower protein intake to any cancer patient or survivor (Muscaritoli M. e., 2021).
- Plant-based diets may compromise bone health—both vegetarians and vegans exhibit lower bone mass density

than omnivores and an increased risk of osteoporosis—which makes these restrictive types of eating behavior quite a bad choice for a breast cancer patient (Li T. Y., 2021). Please read the references instead of defaulting to popular eminence-based trends.
- And regardless of any professional nutrition training whatsoever, most people would not label an Asian vegetarian weight loss plan based on miso, soy sauce, tempeh, and umeboshi as Mediterranean.

Imagine that two doctors in the same city give different diagnoses to identical patients. Then imagine that the exact same doctor makes different therapeutic decisions depending on whether it is morning or afternoon, if he is happy or tired, or if it is Monday rather than Friday. These are examples of what behavioral scientists call noise: variability in judgments that should be identical (Kahneman, 2021). Yet, whereas most don't acknowledge noise even in their own professional field, they completely ignore its existence in such a basic thing as nutrition.

Nonetheless, in Europe, although many hospitalized cancer patients are malnourished or at risk of malnutrition (Arends, 2017), cancer-related malnutrition is under-recognized and mainly undertreated in any way as both professional nutrition knowledge and the use of clinical nutrition and oncology nutrition in the real-world settings are mostly lacking (Caccialanza, 2020). Malnutrition is misclassified in 40% of cases in France (Attar, 2012). A study evaluating 154 hospitals showed that almost half of the patients identified as malnourished received no nutritional support whatsoever (Hébuterne, 2014). In Austria, while a dietician was available in all evaluated hospitals, only 28% of the patients received the referral (Tannen, 2013). In Spain also, only 1/3 of malnourished patients received any kind of nutritional support (Planas, 2016). In Belgium, malnutrition prevalence was 54%, while physicians recognized it only in 16% of cases (Rasschaert, 2024). And the situation is pretty much the same everywhere.

Despite the existing lack of professional nutrition training and the proven inability to recognize or address malnutrition, many healthcare providers think they are entitled to have a say in nutrition simply because they are healthcare providers.

It is true that oncology dietitians are few, and most patients with any cancer barely have access to general dietitians. And maybe because breast cancer patients look more like day-to-day humans rather than some of the cachectic head and neck, esophageal, lung, or pancreatic cancer patients, nowadays, the weight loss industry has moved its focus on slimming them down on autopilot. While the obese breast cancer patients look like fresh meat for its stakeholders, the lack of nutrition professionals is not perceived in clinical settings or in academia, not only because we are few, but because there are over 7 billion eating, buying groceries and cooking experts on Earth. And some are healthcare professionals with no awareness of the actual oncology nutrition guidelines. Consequently, besides the different scoring types subjectively invented, the "Mediterranean" diet—considered as one of the most studied diets in the world—is rather laxly defined, ranging from:

- 3 to 9 portions of vegetables,
- ½ to 2 portions of fruit,
- 1 to 13 portions of cereals (Davis, 2015).

Even the concept of a portion is loosely defined, if at all, as, for instance, the patient's compliance to the DIANA-5 dietary recommendations was assessed only by self-reported 24-hour data collected at baseline, before starting the dietary intervention, and at the end of the first year, without any information about portion size. Authors just invented a restrictive weight loss diet, called it "Mediterranean" and then concluded that "The Mediterranean diet doesn't work in breast cancer."

Numerous studies over several decades imply that following a "Mediterranean" diet can reduce all-cause mortality, cardiovascular diseases, coronary heart disease, myocardial infarction, overall cancer incidence, neurodegenerative diseases, and diabetes (Dinu, 2018). The old ways used to protect Mediterranean people from cardiovascular diseases. However, both the quantity and quality of the present evidence on the many modern versions are highly variable. Many studies do not assess major vascular events, all-cause mortality, or cardiovascular deaths, while serious integrity concerns exist about some of the published data (Liyanage, 2016).

Based on the limited number of studies and their heterogeneity, no convincing evidence exist that such made-up diets decrease blood pressure (Nissensohn, 2016). And despite the large number of published case-control studies on the topic, the quality of the evidence for modest primary cardiovascular prevention is low to moderate, while the evidence for secondary prevention is limited (Rees, 2019). The low-quality data and the many inconsistencies among the methods used for evaluating and defining these fads are hidden behind the health symbol that nowadays got so far from the old Mediterranean ways

The highest adherence to "Mediterranean" diets seems to result in a statistically significant risk reduction for overall cancer mortality and incidence for colorectal, prostate, and aerodigestive cancers, and to statistically nonsignificant changes for breast cancer, gastric cancer, and pancreatic cancer (Schwingshackl L. a., 2014). Further squeezing the evidence, researchers were able to report for the first time a small decrease in breast cancer relative risk (6%) by pooling seven cohort studies (Schwingshackl L. e., 2017). Just that most of the data is of low or very low quality (Morze, 2021).

The modern subjective reinterpretations of the old customs are somewhat of a kakistocracy salad mix of personal opinions sprinkled with up to 8 portions of olive oil per day.

Like taking sugar, flour, and eggs out of a traditional cake, we're pretty much left with a dietetic, artificially sweetened, no-gluten, bland "cake" that would make most Greek grandmothers roll their eyes in disgust as this tastes nothing like the real thing.

None of the old observational or the new randomized trials have anything to do with the traditional gastronomy followed for ages in the Mediterranean countries, as although many are higher in fruits and vegetables than the Western diet, they are not vegetarian, and they are not low fat (Keramaris, 2022).

Greeks traditionally eat lamb.

Umm Ali is an Egyptian classic.

Italian Parmigiano-Reggiano is anything but low-fat.

Jamón is a globally recognized traditional food of Spain.

Contrary to the fact that there is no Mediterranean country where people don't eat meat or dairy since the Seven Country Study, these are considered "non-Mediterranean foods."[3] So, let's look at the available data on meat and dairy in cardiology and oncology settings.

Meat

From a cardiovascular disease prevention point of view, the current literature shows that the association between red and processed meat intake and all-cause mortality or adverse cardiometabolic outcomes is very small, and the evidence is of such low certainty that to even consider it would be an overstretch (Zeraatkar, 2019).

---

[3] https://www.sevencountriesstudy.com/glossary2/mediterranean-diet-score/

Thus, removing cardiovascular disease prevention from the "Mediterranean" diet goals, in oncology settings, some people think that if they don't eat meat, they won't develop cancer, or they'll have higher chances of cure and prevent recurrence because the International Agency for Cancer Research (IARC) classified processed meat as a Group 1 carcinogen.

Processed meat of any color refers to hot dogs, bacon, ham, hamburgers, sausages, and cold cuts.

Red meat refers to lamb, beef, veal, pork, mutton, horse, and goat cooked in any way.

IARC working group concluded that there is limited evidence in humans and inadequate evidence in experimental animals to prove the carcinogenity of red meat. Nevertheless, they ignored the evidence and decided that there is strong potential mechanistic evidence that red meat can be linked to colorectal cancer through N-nitroso compounds, heterocyclic aromatic amines, and heme iron. Thus, they assigned red meat to Group 2A as "probably carcinogenic" contrary to the actual data showing no proof of carcinogenity. Reading the references can help separate eminence-based unprofessional general advice from evidence-based professional personalized recommendations.

There is no connection between unprocessed red meat and N-nitroso compounds, this being an extrapolation from the nitrite used in processed meat. Even for this aspect, the correlation with cancer risk that started from colorectal cancer remains unclear for other cancer localizations (Crowe, 2019). Some epidemiological studies even conclude that "pancreatic cancer risk is lower with higher nitrite intake" (Said Abasse, 2022). Nitrite inhibits Clostridium botulinum growth; it is a taste enhancer and a color-fixing agent, thus making processed meat products cheaper and more appealing.

Although there is no proof that low-nitrite or nitrite-free hot dogs, bacon, or hamburgers remain carcinogenic, N-nitroso compounds can be produced from nitrite, some of which are carcinogenic. And these foods are more difficult to produce, they don't look or taste as good as the nitrite ones, they are higher in salt, and they are more expensive as they have a shorter shelf life (Stoica, 2022).

For unprocessed red meat, studies evaluating the association of heterocyclic amines, polycyclic aromatic hydrocarbons, or benzopyrene (substances formed in meat when fried or overcooked) show only weak correlations with any cancer risk (Kuratko, 2016).

As for the heme iron carcinogenity, in oncology contexts it is important to know that the mechanistic evidence is built on hypothetical *in vitro* scenarios and on animal studies utilizing diets with exaggerations of heme exposure, representing intakes orders of magnitude above the normal dietary consumption of red meat for humans (Kruger, 2018).

Then, the epidemiological studies correlating heme iron intake extrapolated from self-reported food frequency questionnaires with all sorts of health outcomes ignore the fact that heme iron bioavailability differs:

- from male to female in the same species and from muscle to muscle in the same animal (Purchas, 2003),
- for the exact same piece of muscle:
    o by the co-intake of calcium or salt (Kristensen, 2001),
    o by different cooking times, cooking temperatures, and cooking methods (Lombardi-Boccia, 2002).

So, what exactly is correlated with what?

Leaving aside the preclinical and epidemiological assumptions, in clinical settings working with people who already have cancer and are currently under active oncology systemic or local treatments, it is important to keep in mind that non-heme iron from plants has lower bioavailability than heme iron from meat, iron deficiency and iron deficiency anemia being usually more prevalent in vegetarians and vegans (Pawlak, 2018).

And although nowadays we're kind of witnessing a meat-phobia among many eminent scholars, iron deficiency remains the most common global deficiency, being more prevalent in poor populations subsisting on plant-based diets high in compounds that inhibit iron absorption. When high financial resources are on the table, a well-thought vegetarian diet might be adequate for a healthy adult, especially if dietary supplements and iron-fortified foods are used to compensate for the lower non-heme iron bioavailability (Gera T. H., 2012).

However, there is no safety data showing that this is also the case in patients diagnosed with cancers during harsh systemic or local oncology treatments. In oncology settings, cancer itself and the many treatments are associated with an increased risk of anemia (Aapro M. e., 2018), which can be even more prevalent in those with multiple comorbidities (De Franceschi, 2017).

Counteracting anemia in oncology settings can be problematic because iron dietary supplements can worsen the digestive side effects of systemic treatments (Cancelo-Hidalgo, 2013). Additionally, because there is a fine line between iron deficiency and iron overload, supplementation should be done with caution.

The concept of antinutrients seems completely forgotten, unknown or ignored by many.

From an oncology nutrition stance, preventing iron deficiency anemia throughout treatments is not only about the meat intake but mainly about balance. Moving the focus too high on the plant-based side increases the dietary intake of phytates, oxalates, polyphenols, and other plant components that inhibit iron absorption. For instance, excessive intake of whole grains (Ahmed A. M., 2014), whole soybean products (Lynch, 1994), and even the black or green tea so eagerly consumed by many patients after a cancer diagnosis for the contained antioxidants—all these otherwise healthy foods can lower iron bioavailability (Petry, 2014).

Thus, moderation is advised. Balance.

Proper iron intake must be thoroughly evaluated, especially during chemotherapy and surgery, as patients who do not eat enough meat and who consume too many plant foods and teas high in iron absorption inhibiting factors risk worse oncology outcomes as iron deficiency anemia:

- Increases the risk of oncology treatment side effects:
    o During chemotherapy it can worsen fatigue (Harper, 2006) and neuropathy (Tofthagen, 2022). Additionally, it might have an impact on hair loss, although this remains a matter of debate (Raichur, 2017).
    o Preoperative anemia is an independent risk factor for postoperative complications (Sarhane, 2013).
    o Iron deficiency anemia amplifies radiotherapy-induced fatigue (Kowalczyk, 2021).
- Is associated with lower overall survival even in the same clinical stage of breast cancer (Zhang Y. e., 2014).
- Is associated with an increased risk of frailty in the elderly (Palmer, 2018).

When oncology dietitians are missing from the multidisciplinary team, the other healthcare providers may ignore or don't know that there are no oncology settings where low protein intake is professionally recommended, and that anemia must be counteracted by ensuring adequate meat intake and balanced plant-based food intake throughout chemotherapy and surgery. And the "enough meat" is not a 50g, 100g, or 150g preset value abstractly decided based on other people's food frequency questionnaires' answers, but on a thorough clinical evaluation of the individual patient's eating behavior, culture, and sometimes religion, plus at least on the current hemoglobin level, not only on the ferritin which can be biased by concurrent inflammation.

And please ignore for a second the oversimplified working definition that conceptually decided to classify chicken, turkey, and fish as "white meat" for food frequency questionnaire responders to have it easier to answer. Use your own visual perception of color. Look at meat with your eyes!

White meat is fatty meat.

The higher the intramuscular fat in any meat of any species, the whiter the meat. Meat scientists have asked for years for the red vs. white meat epidemiological classification to be removed based on actual muscle histology, but as in the case of BMI, they were and still are ignored in the name of convenience (Seman, 2018). Like, why see the world as it is when one could just decide that it is ~~black~~ red or white?!

The meat of any animal, of any species on the face of the Earth, can be whiter, pinker, or redder based on how sedentary the animal was, a fact we can visually notice when directly inspecting a meat nuance or that we can objectively check with a microscope by assessing the muscle fiber types within that specific piece of meat and the fat within that specific muscle.

Extrapolating the color of meat for an entire species to make it easy for people to answer questionnaires is biological nonsense. Even a wild fish has redder meat than a farmed fish simply because the wild one swam more and thus developed more muscle mitochondria (Keeton, 2017). As there are thin and fat humans, there are thin and fat pigs or thin and fat chickens. And the redder the meat, the leaner it is.

The current IARC consensus is established on low-quality data, a systematic review using the Risk Of Bias In Nonrandomized Studies intervention tool showing that the majority of the studies used as a basis for this consensus had a high risk of bias due to confounding, missing data, and selective outcome reporting (Händel, 2020). But although the information on cancers other than colorectal remains inconsistent to date, the extrapolation has stood tall since 26 October 2015. Why change a perception so clearly established?! Who cares that it contradicts reality as long as it is easy to use, understood and already accepted by the vast majority?

Epidemiological studies evaluate meat carcinogenity by statistically analyzing replies to food frequency questionnaires or 24-hour recalls comparatively between people who declare that they do vs. those who declare they don't eat meat. And even assuming that the recall bias and selection bias are not on the table, we are still left with a question that might cause semantic bias:

What is "cancer" in a questionnaire?

In a questionnaire, "cancer" is a word that collectively defines a multitude of distinctive oncology diagnoses, although even for the same localization, cancers can be completely different from one to another in histology, treatment, and outcome. Nonetheless, the 24-hour recall and the food frequency questionnaires are considered good enough to infer generalizable data.

However, this agreement leads to so many inconsistent results that, to say one way or another looks like a choice built on preset ideas instead of evidence. Consequently, the available epidemiological data is abundant but of low quality (Vernooij, 2019).

For instance, the epidemiological studies on the correlations between red or processed meat intake and kidney cancer risk show that although many studies seem positive, all are weak in magnitude, most are not statistically significant, and associations are attenuated among studies that adjust for confounding factors (Alexander, 2009). Still… newer data suggests that red meat is associated with an increased risk in women. But not in men. And processed meat is detrimental for premenopausal women. But not for men or postmenopausal women (Rohrmann, 2015). And if we remove the mathematical highs and lows, we're kind of left with nothing but airs, as all this is built upon implied excessive intake vs. ascetic avoidance (Ziouziou, 2021).

There is no room for moderation in epidemiology. And in the era where perception has a higher impact than the actual reality, many boldly ignore that correlation does not imply causation. But even the gender-dependent correlation varies so much from study to study that all we're left with are personal interpretations of unverified replies to questionnaires.

Opposite to kidney cancer, excessive red meat intake might be associated with pancreatic cancer risk only in men. And while no biological explanation is offered for any of these mathematic calculations except wild guesses, the available data is inconsistent even for men, as the correlations are found only in case-control studies, while cohort studies report no association (Zhao Z. e., 2017).

Subjective eminence replacing the lack of actual evidence seems common practice worldwide.

The contradiction between case-control vs. cohort results is also present in the case of gastric cancer, with cohort studies showing null results, while case-control ones suggest positive associations (Zhao Z. Z., 2017). And while many keep on forgetting that case-control studies are meant for rare diseases where there is no other option to study potential risk factors, the contradiction happens for ovarian cancers as well, as it does for many others.

Some authors even push the correlation between red and processed meat intake and ovarian cancer risk based on others' case-control studies despite results finding no correlation in their very own cohort data (Kolahdooz, 2010). Nevertheless, the overall evidence shows no correlation between meat intake and ovarian cancer (Gilsing, 2011).

For breast cancer, the popular assumption that red and processed meat intake increases risk also varies from study to study:

- The Black Women's Health Study found no associations between meat, eggs, and dairy intake and breast cancer risk (Genkinger, 2013).
- The MCC-Spain study proposed that breast cancer risk could be reduced by moderating the consumption of well-done or stewed red meat, pan-fried/bread-coated fried white meat, and, especially, processed or cured meat (Boldo, 2018).
- A UK cohort study shows that while red meat consumption was not associated with breast cancer, processed meat consumption was correlated with increased risk only in postmenopausal women. Premenopausal English women can eat all the free-range steak or hot dogs they want, as neither red nor processed meat intake was associated with premenopausal breast cancer in this cohort (Anderson, 2018).

- In contrast, the French NutriNet-Santé cohort found no association between processed meat intake and breast cancer risk but warns about a potential increased risk for red meat both in postmenopausal and premenopausal women (Diallo, 2018).

This contradictory mumbo-jumbo keeps happening from one mixed retrospective and prospective analysis to another (Wu Y. W.-W., 2020). And it is there from the get-go, being core to the self-reported study design. For instance, older studies evaluating measurement error in the 24-hour recalls (Slimani, 2003) and food frequency questionnaires (Kipnis, 2002) used in the European Prospective Investigation of Cancer (EPIC) study by measuring urinary nitrogen excretion as a reference biomarker for protein intake show up to 230% differences between the self-reported and the measured intake.

In 2004-2005, 111 women from the nowadays popular Women's Health Initiative Dietary Modification Trial completed a doubly labeled water protocol (energy biomarker), 24-hour urine collection (protein biomarker), and self-reports of diet (assessed by food frequency questionnaires), exercise, and lifestyle habits. All procedures were repeated after six months (Neuhouser, 2008). This validation study showed that:

- Younger women underreported more than older women.
- Blacks and Hispanics underreported more than Caucasians.
- Obese women underreported energy intake and overreported protein intake.
- Women in the intervention arm underreported dietary intake more than those in the comparison arm; thus, just being a participant in a study can modify how people report things. This begs the question: how are self-reported replies to questionnaires reliable if unverified?

Another validation study that also used measured biomarkers to assess the reliability of dietary self-reports shows that the average differences between self-reported vs. measured intakes for energy, protein, and protein density are:

- 21%, 29%, and 41%, respectively, using food frequency questionnaires (FFQ).
- 26%, 40%, and 36%, respectively, using 24-hour recalls (Freedman, 2014).

Thus, the authors confirmed the existence of systematic bias in dietary self-reports. Nonetheless, unverified dietary intake continues to be ignored, although it is well-recognized (Petersen, 2021). But even when acknowledging the gap between the self-reported and the measured dietary intake, most studies' results are so small that the concept of clinical utility is overly missed. Many systematic reviews and meta-analyses shout from the rooftops that "women who consume red or processed meat have an increased risk of breast cancer" based on data showing that unprocessed red meat associates a relative risk of 1.06, while processed meat one of 1.09 (Farvid M. S., 2018). And 1.06 and 1.09 are mathematically bigger than 1. Still, what is the impact of such a low relative risk on the etiology of a highly multifactorial disease?

The idea that a reduction in processed and red meat intake would result in lower cancer incidence and mortality remains an unproven idea because the evidence is so low-quality due to recall bias, selection bias, semantic bias, residual confounding, and study design limitations, all with an absolute impact on cancer incidence and mortality that is barely there (Han M. A., 2019). And while "further research is warranted" seems like a getaway to defer responsibility for making hypothesis sound like a fact, what oncology nutrition non-professionals are left with to use in clinical practice are subjective reinterpretations of the colorectal cancer extrapolated data, boxed-in together in a retrospective case-control and prospective cohort mess.

In the epidemiologic Utopia, lamb steak, wild turkey pemmican, hot dogs, deep-fried pork meatballs, canned meat, homemade or store-bought liver pates, grass-fed beef stew, free-range chicken soup, barbequed smoked sausages, fast-food fried or crispy baked chicken wings—all are labeled together under the "meat" umbrella.

- But is a Black Angus steak as carcinogenic as hot dogs?
- Are chicken wings fried at home in an air fryer the same as those deep-fried in overused fast-food industry oil?
- Does slow-cooked lamb in the oven have the same metabolic impact as a cheap hamburger?

And although some giraffes only want to see green, while ostriches only want to see gray sand, the scientific truth is that we don't know (Zeraatkar, 2019). All we basically have to make professional recommendations in clinical practice is moderation.

Milk, fermented dairy, and cheese

Unlike meat, where the sky is the limit when it comes to the many opinions but fewer RCTs, there is plenty of RCT evidence on dairy intake showing that there is no apparent risk of harmful effects—irrespective of the content of saturated fat—on a large array of cardiometabolic variables, including lipid-related risk factors, blood pressure, inflammation, insulin resistance, and vascular function, the low-fat guidelines in some countries being unsupported by the scientific literature (Drouin-Chartier, 2016).

And if talking about whole-fat milk used to be sacrilege in cardiology, even mentioning it in oncology settings sometimes seems like blasphemy. This is based either on the hypothesis that milk proteins are carcinogenic or on the one that saturated fats overall are carcinogenic—both mainly extrapolated from the omnipresent but preclinical book titled *The China Study* written by the vegan Collin Campbell, who took Ancel Keys' low-fat recommendations to a whole new level.

The epidemiologic evidence does not support the assumption that these foods are detrimental to breast cancer primary or secondary prevention (Chen L. M., 2019). And while preclinical data should not be used to make professional nutrition recommendations in clinical settings, since this book became so popular among patients diagnosed with cancers, it is important to underline that this book's author published studies showing that carcinogens are more aggressive in the context of low milk protein intake (Campbell, "The effect of quantity and quality of dietary protein on drug metabolism.", 1976) and that we also have others' preclinical data showing that cow milk proteins have anticarcinogenic properties as they:

- Increase overall survival (Engel R. W., 1952).
- Have an anti-mutagenic effect (Van Boekel, 1993).
- Have an anticarcinogenic effect *in vitro* and *in vivo* (Goeptar, 1997).
- Inhibit cancer cell growth and improve immunity (Meisel, 2003).
- Are superior to other dietary proteins for tumor development suppression (Parodi, 2007).
- Decrease cancer onset and proliferation (Duarte D. C., 2011).
- Act as a suppressor of breast tumor growth and metastasis (Bonuccelli, "The milk protein α-casein functions as a tumor suppressor via activation of STAT1 signaling, effectively preventing breast cancer tumor growth and metastasis.", 2012).
- Inhibit angiogenesis (Tung, 2013).
- Have anticarcinogenic and antioxidant effects in metastatic breast cancer, prostate cancer, osteosarcoma, lung, and gastric cancer cell lines (Bielecka, 2022).

I will present in detail the data behind this book in the Veganism Chapter, so let's leave it aside.

Now, probably shocking for people considering milk, dairy, and cheese as non-Mediterranean, food frequency questionnaires self-reported twenty years ago by 280 men and 246 women from Varese, Turin, Florence, and Ragusa exposed that these Italians used to eat "pizza-with-mozzarella" (Fusconi, 2003). And a 2024 visit to the European Institute of Oncology in Milano might currently show that the scientists and clinicians working there still do, while the Milanese pride themselves on having the best pizza in the world, with whole-fat mozzarella.

The subjective "non-Mediterranean foods" working definition of milk, dairy, and cheese used by the low-fat fans since the Seven Country Study was based on the supposed detrimental impact of saturated fats on cardiovascular risk. But there is more than one type of saturated fat.

According to the absence or presence of the double carbon-carbon bond, fats can be classified as saturated or unsaturated. Then, according to the length of the carbon chain within the fatty acid, fats can be classified as short, medium, or long chain. The length of the carbon chain is essential in fatty acid digestion, intestinal absorption, and cellular metabolism. Saturated fats within milk, dairy, and cheese are made of short and medium-length, uneven carbon chain fatty acids, which means that:

- They are the only fats whose digestion starts under the lingual and gastric lipases, thus having a more efficient intestinal absorption even in the case of pancreatic exocrine insufficiency (Turki, 2012).
- Their entrance through both mitochondria membranes does not need carnitine transport (Kerner, 2000).
- They can directly enter the Krebs cycle for complete use—many researchers consider it unfair to generalize

the beneficial metabolism of milk saturated fats to other types of saturated fats (Dawczynski, 2015).

The presence of odd-chain saturated fatty acids in milk is not new evidence (Magidman, 1962). Because of the short and medium length and uneven carbon chain, studies considering this biochemical detail show that higher dairy fat intake is not associated with the presumed increased cardiovascular risk (Liang J. e., 2018). C15:0 and C17:0 fatty acids can be used to distinguish people who eat low-fat vs. whole-fat dairy (Albani, 2016). And just recommending that people eat dairy is insufficient to provide these fatty acids' health benefits. Whole-fat dairy has higher levels of C15:0 and C17:0 saturated fatty acids, which are associated with a decreased risk of cardiovascular disease and all-cause mortality (Trieu, 2021). In light of the evidence, whole-fat milk, dairy, and cheese have a different cardiovascular impact than the one of other dietary sources of saturated fats (Duarte C. e., 2021). Thus, Ancel Keys's recommendation to restrict dairy saturated fat is getting outdated day after day, with the whole-fat dairy intake having no adverse impact on cardiovascular risk (Pokala, 2024).

In regard to breast cancer, one can choose to ignore the different types of saturated fats and simply continue to call them all "saturated fats, and that's that." And it would be at least inconvenient and probably inefficient to give a biochemistry lesson to each participant in a questionnaire-based study. But even in epidemiological studies, low-fat diets are not associated with decreased breast cancer risk, and to increase risk, the overall intake of "saturated fats, and that's that" must be excessive. For instance, a correlation with increased breast cancer risk was found only for an excessive intake of "saturated fats, and that's that" of more than 40% of the total dietary intake—the correlation being valid only in postmenopausal women who didn't use hormone replacement therapy (Thiébaut, 2007).

If, on the other hand, one chooses to no longer consider the "saturated fats and that's that" generalization valid, we even have data showing that the saturated fat in milk has anticarcinogenic, antioxidant, anti-inflammatory, and immunostimulatory properties (Rodríguez-Alcalá, 2017). It is preclinical, but it's there to be further taken into consideration in proper studies. Based on the current epidemiological data available on the metabolic impact of proteins and saturated fats, probiotics, calcium, and vitamin D within milk, fermented dairies, and cheese, there is no professional reason to recommend against their intake neither in general, nor in specific ethnicities (Zang, 2015).

Contrary to popular assumptions, preclinical, epidemiological, and little RCT data show that these foods, traditionally consumed in all Mediterranean countries, associate a reduced risk of breast and colorectal cancer, type 2 diabetes, improved weight maintenance, and improved cardiovascular, bone, and gastrointestinal health (Savaiano, 2021). The correlation between saturated fats and breast cancer risk is controversial because there is no spotlight on moderate intake. What is missed in the way observational studies are reported is that they compare the highest intake with the lowest one while ignoring the middle ground.

Is excess implied upfront to promote subjective ideas contradicted by others' subjective ideas?

And when reality shows that the outcome of the low-fat American recommendation led to more cardiovascular disease and obesity over the years, do we all keep on with the old agreed-upon saga, or do we ask the proposing scientists to take accountability, apologize, and make amends?

While humans' excessive intake is implied and assumed detrimental, the industry's mantra of more is better dietary supplements is gradually built and assumed beneficial.

The "your excess is bad, our excess is better" mindset seems to fuel the fact that nowadays, many healthcare providers and lay people alike ignore that dietary supplements should not replace real foods and specifically recommend the avoidance of entire food categories while relying on dietary supplements to replace their macro- or micronutrients. Thus, in oncology settings, it is important to know that interventional studies on whey proteins, probiotics, calcium, and vitamin D dietary supplements show that:

- Whey protein supplements do not improve any of the tested sarcopenia-linked parameters when compared to whole-dairy foods (Kamińska, 2023).
- Probiotics seem to have a potential role in both the prevention and treatment of breast cancer. However, more clinical studies are needed to elucidate the efficacy and safety of probiotic supplements during oncology treatments (Ranjbar, 2019).
- Some observational and RCT studies of calcium supplementation suggest a potential for cardiovascular harm; thus, calcium supplementation should be used cautiously, striving to achieve the recommended intake from foods (Michos, 2021).
- Infrequent milk consumers have a higher prevalence of vitamin D deficiency (Liu X. A., 2018).
- Dairy consumption is important for proper vitamin D status, even in people taking vitamin D supplements (Levy M. A., 2015).
- A significant and positive correlation between vitamin D status and total intake of dairy products is present even in sunny countries regardless of calcium and/or vitamin D supplementation (Al-Raddadi, 2018).
- Overcorrection can lead to dysregulated vitamin D metabolism, and there is a growing risk of vitamin D toxicity from inappropriate supplementation practices (Taylor P. N., 2018).

- RCTs of the past 100 years show no efficacy of vitamin D supplements in preventing cardiovascular diseases, type 2 diabetes, asthma, respiratory infections, or cancer (Autier, 2017).
- Without objectively proven deficiency, vitamin D supplementation doesn't improve musculoskeletal health (Bolland, 2018), it does not prevent osteoporosis (Reis, 2023), and there is no cardiovascular protection (Virtanen, 2022).
- Supplementing unscreened adults with vitamin D does not reduce all-cause mortality or cancer-specific mortality (Neale, 2022).

According to the law, no one has any legal responsibility for recommending dietary supplements besides the adult who chooses to take these products. These are not medicines. It is our professional responsibility to help the patient make an informed decision based on the actual data instead of on our personal opinions. We know that people whose diets are low in fruits and vegetables, alongside other poor lifestyle choices, have worse health. This is common sense. Recommending the avoidance of food because some correlative studies show that the excessive intake of a particular nutrient naturally found within that food might have a detrimental impact may be interesting to talk about at conferences. But besides the fact that we know that the dairy matrix exerts a beneficial effect more than the sum of its nutrients (Geiker, 2020), applying mathematics to subjective semantics used to assess unverified answers to food frequency questionnaires or 24-hour self-reported recalls ignores human nature.

These built-up theories lack the human experience altogether. Many people would think twice before speaking after enduring chemotherapy or if they knew they'd lose their breast in tomorrow's surgery. Even a man diagnosed with breast cancer would be a bit less talkative before a radical mastectomy.

These epidemiologic correlations have nothing to do with the reality of the Mediterranean area, and they have nothing to do with being two weeks into radiotherapy while everyone keeps throwing contradictory eating advice at you. Financial resources, logistic meals set up during the long days of treatment, emotional eating, mucositis, constipation or diarrhea, the metallic taste, and the exhaustion paralleled with low-quality sleep; all these are overlooked when casually talking about eating in oncology. And while cold mathematics does not delete the complexity of eating behavior, what we all might get from the global pseudo-oncology nutrition salad is lowered compliance due to patients' shame for not being able to apply this or that.

Professional nutrition is not a license to distress other people. Professional nutrition is part of the supportive care needed to help these people have an easier life during treatments with high emotional, social, and financial impacts on their lives.

It is true that obesity and specific unhealthy behaviors like higher alcohol intake, emotional eating, and the yo-yo dieting ping-ponged with the Western fast-food diets low in fruits and vegetables, are associated with an increased risk of cardiovascular diseases, all sorts of different cancers, and premature mortality. The eating pattern associated with an increased cancer risk is specific to highly civilized countries:

- insufficient intake of fruits and fresh vegetables,
- frequent intake of fast food and ready-to-eat products,
- frequent or excessive intake of sweets and soft drinks,
- smoking, sedentariness, excessive alcohol intake, disturbed sleep, and loneliness.

These modifiable behaviors are important to count in when considering primary or secondary cardiovascular disease or cancer prevention, but in the many correlational studies, mutual statistical control is used for the other behaviors to identify independent effects, while in real life, these behaviors coexist. And amid the many academic Utopia vs. reality debates on what a "Mediterranean" diet is or is not, many keep on forgetting that Keys and the other low-fat pioneers from the late 1950s just observed some people living their remote lives. Thus, the biggest stretch of all is the assumption that eating like a peaceful villager would somehow improve the overall health of stressed, sedentary, tired, and lonely people living in big cities.

This was not a diet.

It was a lifestyle with lots of work around the house or in agriculture, which meant regular physical activity, mid-day sleep, which meant adequate rest, and meals cooked at home and eaten together in the family with talks and laughter around the kitchen table, which meant healthier nutritional, emotional, and social life. Happy people may live longer because of factors unrelated to the diet, like family and community satisfaction, while loneliness highly affects health (Fuchsman, 2023).

The physical activity, the siesta, the hospitality, the pure joy of sharing a cookie with your grandma, and the other social aspects of the Mediterranean traditional ways of living as part of a community were lost in translation, though all contribute to a longer, healthier life. And maybe amid the worldwide acculturation, the same happened with people's identities.

Professional oncology nutrition is the traditional Mediterranean way of eating and living together without the modern quotation add-ons: higher in vegetables and fruits, whole grain cereals, legumes, and nuts than the global Western diet but adequately balanced with a moderate intake of lean meat of any species, fish, eggs, whole-fat milk, fermented dairy, and cheese. A feasible diet that can be applied in the long-term needs to focus on food appropriate to each specific culture instead of on paternalistic restrictions. Based on the current evidence, no food category should be excluded in oncology settings.

Chapter 4

Physical activity

The civilized and comfortable lifestyle encourages sedentariness, as working at a desk for 8 hours, driving for 1-2 hours, then sitting on the couch or in front of the TV for 2-3 hours at night, and then sleeping for 6-8 hours, seems to leave little time for physical exercise. To counteract this comfortable, new reality, the World Health Organization cites on autopilot the "strong evidence" that practicing 150-300' of low-moderate intensity physical exercise or 75-150' of higher intensity physical exercises per week decreases the risks for breast, colon, bladder, endometrial, esophageal, kidney, and gastric cancers (WHO, 2018). However, while many embrace popular messages as certain, even for the prevention of breast and colon cancer where evidence looks strongest, this view is not universal.

For instance, the World Cancer Research Fund and the American Institute for Cancer researchers are more circumspect than the WHO, citing only three sites with good enough evidence of a protective effect from physical exercise: breast (but only in postmenopausal women), colon, and endometrial cancers (Clinton, 2020). Across hundreds of epidemiological studies, those with the highest physical activity levels barely achieved a 10%-20% relative risk reduction when compared with the least active ones (McTiernan, 2019). Thus, here we stumble again on eminence-based contradictory opinions, many ignoring both the high risk of bias of questionnaire-based studies and the little impact of point-zero-something relative risks.

The guidelines are based on systematic reviews, meta-analyses, and analyses of pooled data from observational studies where physical activity is self-declared and unverified in any way, exercise being broadly defined, with little focus on its intensity as compared to the individual's level of fitness, and with assumed continued practice after the completion of the questionnaire.

For instance, one of the studies evaluating exercise's impact on cancer risk is the PLCO prospective screening study (Prostate, Lung, Colon, and Ovary), which started in 1993 and finished in 2017. Blood specimens from the screened participants, oral cell DNA from controls, and histology slides from cancer cases were collected.

Participants completed a baseline questionnaire at recruitment covering health status, risk factors, and a dietary questionnaire. The intervention arm received screening, while the control received only usual care. More than 12,000 participants were enrolled in the pilot phase, which started in 1993 and was completed in 1994, with enrollment exceeding 144,500 in 2000. Physical exercise was evaluated based on the question, "How many hours do you spend in vigorous activities, such as swimming, brisk walking, etc.?" to which participants could answer by choosing one of the six preset options: "none"; "less than 1 hour per week"; "1 hour per week"; "2 hours per week"; "3 hours per week"; and "$\geq$4 hours per week" (Gohagan, 2000).

To approximate the US definition of vigorous exercise as $\geq$ 75 minutes per week, 66% of participants were classified as exercisers ($\geq$ 1h per week) and 34% as non-exercisers (< 1h per week). But…

First, "Exercisers were more likely to report fewer pack-years of smoking, have lower BMI, and were less likely to have arthritis, chronic bronchitis, diabetes, emphysema, and hypertension." Thus, does physical exercise per se decrease cancer risk, or does the overall healthy lifestyle—that includes physical exercise among other healthy behaviors—decrease cancer risk?

Second, in this article, the detail that self-reported physical exercise "is reliable and strongly correlates with the objective assessment made with accelerometers" is assumed as fact based on two quoted studies:

- One performed on 46 women that evaluated self-reported light-intensity sitting, light-to-moderate intensity standing, and walking in comparison to an accelerometer measurement, concluding that the self-reports are "reasonably accurate" (Ainsworth, 1999). How authors got from the original "reasonably accurate" to the "reliable and strongly correlates" only they know.
- One performed on 125 middle school students that had nothing to do with the age category of the PLCO cohort actually concluded the exact opposite: "The preset questions underestimate moderate physical activity and overestimate the vigorous one. The use of accelerometry for physical activity surveillance seems to be indicated. At the minimum, new questions demonstrating greater validity are needed" (Troped, 2007).

What relevance does this one-time, unverified self-report to a vague question with preset answers to choose from have at the time of enrollment if the study design is based on reinterpretation of studies with different age categories, extrapolated to match a preset point of view that contradicts these studies' actual conclusions? And what relevance does it have years later? What relevance does it have even one month later?

This is important as if you'd ask people about their exercise habits at the beginning of January when many vividly start their New Year's resolutions, or if you'd ask the exact same questions at the beginning of February when many already gave up, you'd get completely different answers. So, does this data have any weight?

The answer might probably explain the puzzling results (Lavery, 2024), showing that physical exercise:

- lowers the risk of head and neck (31%), lung (23%) and breast cancers (11%),
- has no correlation with colon, gastric, bladder, endometrial, and renal cancers,
- increases the risk of prostate cancer (13%) and melanoma (15%).

As many would say, the authors concluded that the increased melanoma risk makes sense as highly active people spend a lot of time in the sun. But no one asked anyone if they exercised outside or indoors or if they wore sunscreen or not. This was just an assumption that had nothing to do with this study's participants. And the men of the world considering prostate cancer prevention received no explanation, as a plausible one could not be conceived.

In the little available free time, many busy clinicians got so used to reading only the abstracts instead of the whole study data that they now ignore on autopilot that there is little evidence for efficacy to most of the cancer prevention epidemiological propaganda.

It seems like guidelines are built on good intentions, as health policymakers want to somehow make people do this or that, regardless of the available data. And they sound so healthy and nice!

How much of a difference can physical exercise make in the prevention of diseases with such complex etiology as cancers is kept aside, as the lack of evidence is replaced by eminence and popularity.

What the few people who manage to keep up their New Year's resolutions all year long do is basically keep it small, doable, and as simple as possible within their individual means. I've worked with people trying to improve their diet and lifestyle for the past decade, and what I can say after assisting thousands of cancer patients in improving their lives is that change is hard. Self-trust is built on small wins, while the big, ego-driven goals are often self-defeating. How many of us have 300' a week to exercise? And how is the statement "exceeding the upper limit of 300' is optimal" accurate if 150' vs. 300' barely makes a difference? For instance, the postmenopausal breast cancer relative risk reduction is 6% at 150' of physical activity per week and 10% at 300' per week (Matthews C. E., 2020). Does a 4% relative risk reduction have enough clinical impact to say that "more is better"?

For instance, doing 250 squats with an Apple watch on takes about 10'.

If one does this effort five times per week, it doesn't matter because it only takes 50'? I dare people who say that doing < 1h of sports per week is insufficient to have a positive impact on health to research it on their own health by doing 5 x 250 squats per week for at least one month.

And imagine you're one of the 20,120 in the PLCO study reporting < 1h of sport per week, and although you managed to regularly squeeze in between your family and your busy professional day-to-day life a 20' run twice a week, some people would equal your physical and many times high logistical effort to zero. Would this motivate you to do more, or would you just gradually lose your drive to do it and give up on the whole exercise hurdle? What is the societal consequence of telling people that doing less than 1h of sports per week equals zero? How many postmenopausal 60-something women would do more than that? And how many sedentary healthcare provider men would start exercising if $p<0.001$ data formally endorsed by the American Cancer Society points out that exercise is associated with increased prostate cancer risk?

Is cherry-picking the positive statistics while ignoring the negative ones, science or politics?

Abstract epidemiology is offensive, and many fight back the offense by doing even more nothing.

Like a displeased parent feeling entitled to hit his child for doing only the little of his homework that he knew how to do, amid the "more is better" mindset meant to slap back sedentariness, people are boxed in demotivating categories to allow statisticians to do their calculus and epidemiologists to publish their studies, with no responsibility for the societal impact and with little focus on the main benefit of physical exercise: avoiding primary (age-related) and secondary (disease- and/or treatment-related) sarcopenia.

Exercise improves muscle quality in people at risk for sarcopenia and sarcopenic obesity (Ramírez-Vélez, 2021). This is also true in oncology settings (Cao A. e., 2022). And this is true even for a single resistance training session a week (Santos, 2019). A journey of 1000 miles starts with a single step; thus, any little amount of physical activity counts.

For instance, unlike other types of cancers, breast cancers are not hypermetabolic per se and do not associate secondary sarcopenia, cachexia, or weight loss. However, some of the breast cancer treatments do have a muscular detrimental impact: chemotherapy, aromatase inhibitors, and salpingo-oophorectomy.

During these systemic treatments and after the risk-reducing surgery, besides having a proper protein intake, physical exercise is the second mandatory factor important to maintaining muscle mass and, therefore, metabolism. Without these two, fat gain is ensured as the muscle protein synthesis/ muscle protein degradation ratio leans into the treatment-induced degradation side (Papadopetraki, 2023). However, without a body composition measurement, people see this as plain weight gain, although this is mainly not based on eating more but on muscle loss due to either too low protein intake, sedentariness, or both.

Sarcopenic obesity prevention should start from the beginning of neoadjuvant chemotherapy, which is the first treatment that associates muscle loss and subsequent metabolism decrease during many breast cancer patients' treatment trajectory.

From a professional nutrition point of view, preventing or correcting sarcopenia is all about ensuring that the patients have and are able to digest the higher protein intake required to keep the muscle protein synthesis/ muscle protein breakdown ratio as balanced as possible throughout this treatment. And what non-nutrition healthcare providers throwing low-protein diets at cancer patients during chemotherapy seem not to know or choose to ignore is that:

- Without proper protein intake, this ratio cannot be balanced by sport alone (Koopman R. , 2007), this being even more important in the case of the anabolic resistance present in the elderly (Zaromskyte, 2021) and in patients with cancer (Pérez-Bilbao, 2023).
- Without physical exercise, this ratio cannot be balanced by nutrition alone (Witard, 2021).
- With proper physical exercise and protein intake, this ratio cannot be maintained under energy deficit even in

trained healthy women with high protein intake (Oxfeldt, 2023); thus, caloric restriction should be judiciously weighted before being recommended to patients at risk for primary or secondary sarcopenia.
- Stressing the patient to lose weight instead of encouraging proper nutrition and exercise within each individual's means is useless and adds to the stress already built in the oncology settings, potentially increasing the fear of recurrence (Bentley, 2024).

Traditionally, physical activity has been classified as either "resistance" or "aerobic" exercise, the main difference being that aerobic exercise (repeated low-intensity muscle contractions) mainly results in a shift toward more muscle fibers with greater oxidative capacity. In contrast, resistance exercise (higher-intensity muscle contractions) induces muscle hypertrophy. In reality, there is considerable overlap between these didactic definitions, results specific to each fitness level, regularity of practice, individual movement intensity, rest between sets, and overall training duration (Kumar V. e., 2009).

Resistance exercises like squats, lunges, sit-ups, and so on—performed only with the body weight ± dumbbells or other free weights, or resistance bands—are considered the most effective for preventing or counteracting sarcopenia during breast cancer systemic treatments with muscular side effects (McGovern, 2022), the earlier the start of training and oncology nutrition intervention the higher the efficacy (Jang, 2023). And it is not only about muscle loss. Resistance training practiced during chemotherapy also increases muscle strength and lean body mass while decreasing adiposity (Padilha, 2017).

However, many patients feel ill or fatigued during the first few days after chemotherapy administration, so if one must choose between sedentariness (maximum muscular damage) and resistance exercise (maximum muscular protection) in such cases, one can always choose moderation: aerobic exercises

(Adams S. C., 2016). Combining resistance training with aerobic training seems to be the most effective way to decrease body fat (Liang Z. e., 2023) and reduce fatigue (Medeiros Torres, 2022), while resistance training improves sleep and mood (Maric, 2024). Thus, whenever possible, patients should be encouraged to practice both.

Besides maintaining metabolism by protecting muscle mass, sleep, and mood, aerobic exercises like walking, cycling, swimming, step aerobics, skating in the park, or dancing in the living room during chemotherapy:

- Prevent weight gain (Li X. e., 2024).
- Prevent cardiotoxicity (Tsai Y.-L. e., 2023).
- Prevent neuropathy (Nuñez de Arenas-Arroyo, 2023).
- Are associated with better cognitive function (Salerno, 2021).
- Reduce anxiety and depression (Lee J. a.-G., 2020).
- May be the best nonpharmacologic intervention for chemotherapy-related cognitive impairment in breast cancer patients (Liu Y. e., 2023).

However, in day-to-day clinical practice, many oncologists consider that supportive care means prescribing supplements, ignoring physical exercise, and having no idea that the main oncology nutrition recommendation is about the protein intake being high enough to counteract breast cancer treatment-induced sarcopenia.

Consequently, most patients eat whatever and remain as sedentary as before, both during the chemotherapy months and during the years of antiestrogenic treatment, gradually gaining weight because of the muscle loss and metabolic decrease generated by the lack of supportive care.

Then, the ovarian function suppression—either from chemotherapy in the cases where this happens or from the gonadotropin-releasing hormone analogs—comes with all the usual side effects of menopause that can be improved by the regular practice of physical exercise (Capel-Alcaraz, 2023). Symptoms happen at a hastier pace after salpingo-oophorectomy, though. Weight gain, vasomotor symptoms, sexual dysfunction, bone loss, mood and sleep disturbances, and, at times, lowered cognitive functioning or anxiety abruptly become part of these women's lives after the risk-reducing surgery (Nebgen, 2023). People are not alive only because they're not dead, and they don't die only from breast, ovarian, or serous endometrial cancer. Thus, offering a risk-reducing salpingo-oophorectomy to a breast cancer patient or a healthy BRCA 1/2 mutation carrier without proper supportive care may be a prescription for an alive walking dead with worsened obesity, osteoporosis, cardiovascular disease, diabetes, dementia, and depression (Hassan, 2023).

Neoadjuvant endocrine treatment has become an option for some patients with luminal breast cancers, and although the overall metabolic impact is not as high as the one of chemotherapy, the detrimental muscular impact is there, especially for aromatase inhibitors. Unlike chemotherapy, which adds to the muscular impact of the digestive, neurologic, hematologic, and cardiologic side effects, aromatase inhibitors differ by adding to the muscular impact of osteopenia (or osteoporosis) and arthralgia. The side effects of endocrine treatments are frequent in patients but underestimated or ignored by the system, leading to the poor treatment adherence we all know compromises outcomes.

Besides other pharmacological and non-pharmacological supportive care needed to manage these side effects of the antiestrogenic treatments (Dos Santos, 2021), physical exercise can improve the quality of life of these patients by:

- contributing to weight management (Park S.-H. M., 2019),
- lowering chronic pain (Boing, 2020),
- reducing fatigue (Hall, 2022),
- improving sleep disturbances (McGrorry, 2023), and
- recovering cardiometabolic health (Cheng, 2024).

Sarcopenic obesity initiated after diagnosis if sedentary during neoadjuvant chemotherapy or antiestrogenic treatment is sometimes aggravated by the fact that some breast cancer surgeons contraindicate physical exercise either short-term after surgery or long-term as a way to prevent lymphedema in breast cancer patients with axillary dissection.

For the short-term sedentariness prescribed by most breast cancer surgeons, it is important to know that even five days of muscle disuse substantially lowers muscle protein synthesis even in healthy young people with proper protein intake by anabolic resistance to protein ingestion (Wall, 2016). Thus, the 1–2-month post-surgery period, when patients are usually advised to avoid physical exercise, amplifies the neoadjuvant chemotherapy secondary sarcopenia in those with no access to supportive care.

The surgical scars must be protected until they are completely healed, but even during the first days following surgery: patients can take a walk, take the stairs instead of the elevator, or perform lower body exercises.

For the long-term sedentariness still prescribed by some breast cancer surgeons, it is important to know that there are many RCTs performed on patients with axillary dissection showing that the normal use of both arms for household activities and practicing symmetrical physical exercises does not increase the risk of breast cancer secondary lymphedema (BCRL):

- Upper-body resistance exercises do not increase swelling, discomfort, pain, heaviness, or tightness in the BCRL-affected patients (Cormie, 2013).
- There is no difference regarding seroma formation or dehiscence between patients performing exercises daily at home beginning on postoperative day 1 and those who began the exercises after the drains' removal (Petito, 2014).
- Progressive resistance training improves physical functioning and reduces the risk of BCRL (Cheema, 2014).
- Resistance exercise is safe after axillary dissection and does not generate BCRL (Keilani, 2016).
- Patients with BCRL can safely practice resistance exercises without worsening lymphedema or related symptoms. However, there is insufficient evidence to support or refute the current clinical recommendation to wear compression garments during training (Singh B. e., 2016).
- Patients with breast cancer at risk for BCRL can safely lift weights during upper body resistance exercises without causing lymphedema. Some studies reported that the volume of the lymphedema-affected arm was significantly more reduced in the weightlifting group than in the control group (Wanchai, 2019).
- Resistance training does not have a negative effect; on the contrary, it potentially decreases risk (Hasenoehrl, 2020). Still, more research is needed to say that physical exercise prevents BCRL.

Moreover, since many patients continue to avoid physical exercise during the radiotherapy that frequently follows breast cancer surgery, and since both radiotherapy and axillary surgery co-increase lymphedema risk, it is important to inform them that doing sports during radiotherapy is important also for reducing this treatment's associated fatigue (Lipsett, 2017).

And regardless of the therapeutically required type of breast cancer surgical treatment or radiotherapy administration, obesity and sedentariness remain some of the most important patient-related factors that can aggravate breast cancer treatment secondary lymphedema. Thus, physical exercise is beneficial for patients with or without axillary dissection since:

- The effect of manual lymphatic drainage remains unclear (Müller, 2018).
- The use of intermittent pneumatic compression devices remains controversial due to their adverse effects, including the recurrence of edema and potential lymphatic structure damage due to high-pressure application (Tran K. a., 2018).
- There is insufficient evidence for any pharmacologic therapy for patients with BCRL (Walker J. e., 2022).

Healthy persons can practice physical exercise without being supervised by physical therapists if they know how to perform the movements correctly. In the case of breast cancer patients under active treatment administration and breast cancer survivors, however, it is generally advised that physical exercise would best be performed under specialized supervision (Brown J. C., 2012).

Yet, although many healthcare providers seem to agree that physical exercise is important to counteract the various consequences of oncology treatments, clinical reports show low referral rates to physical therapy (Stout, 2021). And since most breast cancer treatment centers don't have a physical therapist and most patients don't get a rehabilitation referral, they should be supervised by whom?!

In real clinical practice, many patients during active breast cancer treatments remain as sedentary as before the diagnosis, even some of those who participated in physical exercise trials gradually getting back to being sedentary post-intervention. Some patients stop training because they don't have the time, money, or knowledge needed to do it at the high level they perceive they should. Others interpret the temporary recommendation to "avoid physical exercise" after surgery as a professional prescription for long-term sedentariness. Others, like most of us, have many competing activities they ought to do in the limited amount of free time needed for sports activities. Some don't even start because of a too-long commute to the training facility, while no one has told them they can efficiently train in the privacy of their own home (Gollhofer, 2015).

How do we fix it?

If we have enough humility to set the bar properly low, then any of us can be better tomorrow.

If the bar is set too high by ego-driven expectations, most people will not even try.

The benefits of practicing physical exercise only occur if consistent training becomes a lifestyle habit, not if the scared patient runs a marathon and then lies down for a year. 75, 150, and 300 are just numbers that help no one with nothing in the long run, except maybe to publish health guidelines that are mainly ignored even by the people who make them. The key to doing sports long-term is to start with something you can enjoy doing day by day. Your favorite music or training with friends can help build and maintain the habit of practicing sports for life. Do something so easy to practice and so simple to integrate into the daily schedule that you'd have no excuse not to do it. Waltz, ping-pong, kiteboarding, shadow boxing, and golf are just some of the many physical exercises with a positive health impact. Everyone can do any little amount of any physical activity they're able and prefer to do, as even walking counts (Wang P. e., 2022).

You don't like squats? Don't do squats.

It doesn't have to be resistance training because it's the best of the best.

It doesn't have to be yoga because it's the new breast cancer hype.

Should've, would've, and could've are empty words.

Shorter lengths of time, longer lengths of time… if you like it enough to do it, it doesn't really matter. And this is not about being a patient or not; this is about human nature. Prescribing the best while ignoring the rest brings no real-world benefit as people live in their own lives instead of the Utopia where we all have the time and are in the mood for all of the many healthy behaviors. "This is the best!" "Strive for that!" or "Try the other!" are just opinions, frequently unsolicited, frequently ignored, and frequently not practiced even by the people who promote them. As Professor Dan Ariely likes to say:

"We all are wonderful people in the future. We really are. Tomorrow."

BEHAVIORS THAT AMPLIFY MUSCLE LOSS

Chapter 5
Non-compliance

There is a huge gap between real clinical settings and well-crafted academic settings, kind of like the St. Gallen consensus conference where what we're supposed to do is built on the assumption that all resources are available. Although this conference is high up on top of my preferences for the geek that I am due to the high quality of the lectures, the consensus part frequently conflicts with clinical reality as, sadly, all resources are often not that available. Even most of the experts who vote don't have access to all the agents they officially assume are available, while some of them seem to have so little experience outside clinical trials that they may not be aware of how things work in reality.

The assumption of resource availability in rose-tinted glasses remains a cozy idea, while real-life compliance with any "should" remains resource-dependent. Outside conference walls, behind the absence of a behavior, there is always a lack of resources. And while money is often part of the problem, resources are not only financial.

Time can be an issue.

Religion can be an issue.

Social support can be an issue.

Properly trained human resources can be an issue.

Access to appropriately equipped treatment facilities can be an issue. Rigid mindset, miscommunication, being treated in another country, having a sick child, extremes of age, personality disorders, cognitive dissonance, anxiety, depression, or loneliness can be an issue.

If we expect anyone to accept chemotherapy or the required surgery, do the recommended radiotherapy, take their medications, do the proper follow-up for 5-10 years after the diagnosis, eat right, do the advised physical exercise, and recover mentally and emotionally, then time, money, social support, knowledge, personal resilience, and even peace need to be on the table.

Any discussions about what should be expected from the people working in oncology settings and about what should be expected from the people treated in oncology settings should start with the acknowledgment that we're all people and that we're in this together. Unlike Utopia, where conditions are perfect, and everything is already provided, in real clinical settings, there are two types of treatments:

- **PROCEDURES done to the patient** – where we get nothing if the people working in oncology settings don't make the proper recommendations and if the people treated in oncology settings don't accept the recommendation, like surgery, radiotherapy, or intravenous chemotherapy.
- **BEHAVIORS done by the patient** – where we get nothing if the people working in healthcare don't make the proper recommendations and if the people with the cancer diagnosis don't apply the recommendation, like

practicing breast cancer screening, taking the antiestrogenic medication or capecitabine, and practicing physical activity, sleep hygiene, smoking cessation, psychotherapy, and oncology nutrition.

Many see this only as "the people working in healthcare should make recommendations," forgetting or disregarding the word "proper." The basis of "proper" is for each of us to do our own part, each in our own area of expertise. Casually stepping outside of each area of expertise is frequent in oncology, though. Thus, for increased efficacy and the health and well-being of all of us, it is important to acknowledge that this well-meant mindset has at least three issues.

First, we're all human.

In breast cancer settings, the focus is on patients' non-compliance to antiestrogenic treatment administration, as this behavior is associated with lower overall survival (Eliassen F. M., 2023). Non-compliance hits us hard in nutrition, psychotherapy, and physical therapy. Many patients start supportive care interventions with high determination, then kind of do it for a while, then pendule between falling off the wagon and getting back on, in a never-ending repetition compulsion that gets them nowhere (Artene, 2018). Thus, actually obtaining and maintaining the expected supportive care benefits simply because supportive care was prescribed is a bit more complicated than what most would assume. And it's not about us. And it's not about them. It's about being human.

And sometimes, human nature doesn't give a heck about others feeling ill during chemotherapy. Data from the Global Oncology Monitor on 45,324 patients treated with chemotherapy in France, Germany, Italy, Spain, and the UK shows that physicians don't prescribe antiemetic medications based on MASCC/ESMO guidelines but based on their subjective perceptions of the emetic risk, oncologists' compliance to antiemetic guidelines being roughly 15%. In this real-world study, way away from the shiny conference rooms where everyone seems so nice and dandy, 12% of patients received no antiemetics whatsoever during chemotherapy. And, mathematically, 12% might seem quite a decent number. But humans are not numbers, and 12% of 45,324 equals 5438 people who experienced nausea and vomiting during chemotherapy simply because (Aapro M. e., 2021).

Besides prescribing or not prescribing supportive care, many physicians try to use reason, assuming it is enough for patients to understand our "why" to just apply it. This thinking ignores that most people—healthy or sick—don't just do what they're told to do based on scientific data pointing out that their behavior is wrong. Nevertheless, providing educational materials is the most common intervention already implemented to improve adherence. According to the available efficacy data though, knowledge alone doesn't work to change a behavior in the long-term (Ekinci, 2018).

Miscommunication contributes to non-compliance, and it runs both ways:

- **Miscommunication from the healthcare provider's side** is still an issue:
  o Among clinicians who don't even intend to apply it, the lack of shared decision-making is associated with lower patient compliance (Montagna E. e., 2021).
  o Among clinicians who intend to apply it, implementation is sometimes limited by the subjective understanding of shared decision-making (Savelberg, 2019).
- **Miscommunication from the patient's side** also is still an issue:
  o Women < 40 and ≥ 80 years old (Dragvoll, 2022) and men with early-stage breast cancers (Sauder,

2020) sometimes do not understand the risk/benefit ratio of antiestrogenic treatment or radiotherapy after breast-conserving surgery.

- Some young patients with good prognosis really want to have kids and emotionally shut down when the issue is abruptly contraindicated by the medical oncologist. And this is not rare. Surveys show that 46.9% of oncologists never consulted the available international guidelines on pregnancy after breast cancer (Lambertini, 2018).
- Some patients find it difficult to express their doubts and worries about the treatment recommendation received during the tumor board (Savelberg, "Does lack of deeper understanding of shared decision making explains the suboptimal performance on crucial parts of it? An example from breast cancer care.", 2019).
- Some people are non-compliant by nature. An analysis performed on 21,255 breast cancer patients showed that those non-compliant with any medication before the cancer diagnosis have twice the risk of being non-compliant with antiestrogenic treatment administration (Neugut, 2016).
- While some simply do not share their private logistic factors that impede compliance, a recent systematic review showed an average non-compliance of 28.3% to the scheduled radiotherapy, roughly leading to 1/3 of patients having increased recurrence and mortality (Suryanegara, 2022). But did the patient not do the recommended radiotherapy because they didn't want to, because they thought it would be of no benefit, or because they, for instance, lived so far from the radiotherapy center that the daily commute made them decide not to do it from the get-go? Simply observing non-compliance without trying to understand the reasons behind this behavior is inefficient in changing it for the better.

On our side, we need to remember we're not the only experts in the room.

People diagnosed with cancer are among the experts in the room. They are the ones knowing their own resources and shortcomings at the expert level. They know who they are. We don't. Each person is a unique individual with unique positive and negative body and mind traits and unique life circumstances. Expecting we all speak English simply because it's mainly spoken doesn't change the fact that at home, we speak our mother tongue. Assuming that adopting the king's language will make the world a better place is a convenient assumption that doesn't wipe out either that diversity helped us survive as a species or that keeping each personal identity has a positive mental and social impact.

If all a grandmother or a nanny diagnosed with breast cancer can do as physical exercise is to play with the children in the park, we should encourage that. And if a young, ambitious CEO treated with axillary dissection wants to participate in a dragon boat paddling competition, we should encourage that as well by providing the proper kinetic knowledge necessary for her to do it. Still, many healthcare providers project their subjective ideas onto patients in areas where they know little about. Opinionating is not professional at any level, but it is highly human. Thus, it's highly practiced.

Giving a heck about self or others and having the courage, the willingness, or the openness to speak up, the health literacy, the trust, the time, and the financial status and social support can be non-compliance risk factors. However, treatment side effects are the most commonly reported patient-related reason for low adherence or treatment discontinuation, with most non-compliant patients choosing it because of vasomotor symptoms, sexual dysfunction, weight gain, sleep disturbances, and cognitive decline that subsequently mess up their lives (Goldberg, 2024).

Affected patients are frequently met by healthcare system-related factors that ignore their symptoms or offer no solution:

- Follow-up care by a general practitioner (Cahir, 2015), frequently with little understanding of what the breast cancer experience actually implies at a human level (Paranjpe, 2019).
- Insufficient information and support even from the treating healthcare professionals (Clancy, 2020).

Is feeling ill from a treatment not feeling ill because it's objectively justified?

How are patients supposed to be long-term compliant with no means to manage side effects?

Pointing the finger at patients' non-compliance as a cause for decreased overall survival seems valid. However, data shows that physicians' non-compliance is as prevalent as the patients', with about 42.5% of therapeutic decisions being based on subjective perceptions, personal preferences, lack of knowledge, or subjective decisions instead of guidelines (Nino de Guzman, 2020). It is true that there are differences between ESMO and NCCN guidelines (Zagouri, 2015), but many are unaware of these differences and basically ignore even the ones official in their own geographical area.

And while it takes two to tango, patients' non-compliance decreases their own survival, while physicians' non-compliance decreases patients' survival (Ricci-Cabello, 2020).

Some well-meant older medicine professors are not aware that about half of patients don't take their medications or that about half of physicians don't follow guidelines. And when they realize that this is actually happening, they try to somehow cover it up by overworking themselves.

Exactly like fathers who try their best to protect and provide as much as possible for their families, they inspire us to become better through accountability and positive personal examples. But good intentions and trying to be the best you can possibly be to provide all the care you understand is needed for your patient doesn't change either that you're human too, or that these are different healthcare professions than your own, with as many professional nuances as your own. No one can do it all without getting themselves sick.

On the opposite side of the father-like medical figures who forget to put their own oxygen mask first, there are the bullies who managed to get to powerful positions in medicine and who disrespect the other physicians, nurses, and healthcare professionals. Supportive care professionals are usually less exposed to this entitled attitude because the classical medical system was mainly built for physicians and nurses. Many physical therapists, psychologists, and dieticians do not even consider working in hospitals, directly choosing private practice. Occasionally, nurses may feel at these abusers' mercy as most don't have the guts or the position to call them out, choosing to change jobs or professions because of the unprofessional mistreatment some think they must tolerate.

Domineering, controlling, dismissive and divalike healthcare providers are part of the causes of lowered patients' trust in allopathic medicine.

Abuse in healthcare is defined by patients' subjective experiences characterized by lack of care (Brüggemann, 2012). Racism, unprofessional behavior, non-personalized recommendations, invasion of privacy, shaming or embarrassment, information withholding, and abuse of power are the quoted reasons that managed to destroy some patients' trust so badly that they no longer want to have anything to do with the allopath system (Mazur, 2024).

All of us look kind of bad when someone in our family acts like an entitled prick, but all of us are not entitled pricks. And, in oncology, patients are best treated within the knowledge of allopath medicine.

Just that, additionally to the bullies, there are those who create animosities, distrust, and unnecessary expenses deep within the healthcare system by overtreating patients. For instance, Choosing Wisely was created to promote patient-physician conversations about unnecessary medical investigations and treatments as, by some estimates, over $760 billion are pointlessly wasted each year, accounting for approximately 25% of the total US healthcare spending (Shrank, 2019). Conversely, the rates of contralateral prophylactic mastectomy in patients with unilateral low-risk breast cancers remain high in the US (Wang T. A., 2020). Some of these surgeons quote the patient's request for body symmetry as a reason for this therapeutically unnecessary surgery (Pender, 2023). Others continue to promote mastectomy to younger patients as a safer treatment than breast conservation despite data showing that larger surgery does not equal better outcomes even though young age is an independent risk factor for increased local recurrence:

- After the introduction of molecular subtypes and improved systemic treatments, local control and overall prognosis have improved significantly in young women too, with the expected risk of local recurrence at ten years after breast-conserving treatment decreasing from 14.2% in 1997 to 4.8% in 2010 (Botteri, 2017).
- An almost decade-old meta-analysis of 22,598 patients younger than 40 with T1-T2, N0–N+, and M0 breast cancers shows better overall survival for patients treated with breast conservation and whole breast radiotherapy when compared with those treated with mastectomy (Vila, 2015).

Others continue to promote mastectomy to patients with early breast cancers older than 50 (De la Cruz Ku, 2022), while others underline that the overall certainty of the data showing that breast-conserving surgery plus radiotherapy improves cancer-specific survival when compared with mastectomy alone is very low (Rajan, 2024). Nevertheless, a long time ago, Black Cady used to say that in the world of surgical oncology, "biology is king, selection of cases is queen, and the technical details of surgical procedures are the princes and princesses of the realm who frequently try to overthrow the king and queen, usually to no long-term avail, although with some temporary apparent victories" (Cady, 1997).

Although for the past four decades, data continued to show that mastectomy brings no benefit over breast conservation in patients with early breast cancers, some surgeons act like princes and princesses who got so used to the mastectomy mantra that they refuse to give it up. Consequently, the overtreatment is still proposed to women eligible for breast conservation, who are convinced they will look and be better after prophylactic surgery (Montagna G. a., 2020). Is the rise of contralateral prophylactic mastectomy in patients who don't even meet the criteria for unilateral therapeutic mastectomy, surgeons' non-compliance, surgical treatment led by patient's anxiety, or both? And, in cases where this is on the table, is anxiety treated with surgery?

Second, all humans go to hell when running on empty.

And in oncology settings, we're talking about more than just physical fatigue. It's lassitude, a physical and mental weariness that can burn anyone out. Sadly, both when it comes to treatment non-compliance and when it comes to lassitude, the double standard seems kind of locked in, with many focusing on patients only, forgetting that healthcare providers get physically and emotionally tired, too.

Most healthcare providers want to help patients, and most patients want to be educated on how to contribute to their own healing. But the road to hell seems literally paved with all of our good intentions, some people taking on their plate more than one could possibly chew without having the proper professional training for the many things they try to add extra to their profession.

Some of the healthcare professionals who not only choose to do more than they professionally should but are frequently imposed by the system to do more than their profession are oncology nurses. In eight hospitals in Catalonia, Spain, virtually all oncology nurses participating in a study perceived the need for emotional management training, as compassion fatigue lowered their empathy while increasing their anxiety and desire to leave their units or change their profession (Arimon-Pagès, 2019). Including nurses in the decision-making processes regarding their own professional practice is crucial to reducing their turnover intentions (Marques-Pinto, 2018). How are non-psychology healthcare providers supposed to be professional and empathetic with patients and also find ways to avoid burnout if they're required to do more than their profession and are not trained in emotional management? And how professional is it to ask people with no academic training in psychotherapy, physical therapy, or nutrition to provide all these healthcare services on top of their professional duties just because they're there?

The old physician-nurse dyad is still the main course on the table in hospitals as weight gain, sedentariness, smoking, substance use or non-substance use addictions, loneliness, or disturbed sleep are secondary health issues. Although both of these types of healthcare providers have little formal education in supportive care, many try to compensate for it by doing their best to cover up the holes within the medical system with popular dietary supplements or with casual physical training, psychology, and nutritional suggestions.

The gap between what is elegantly presented at conferences and real-world clinical practice seems at times as huge as China, making many clinicians roll their eyes when another academic colleague comes to enlist how things should run in Utopia, where all resources are available. In the real world, when any of these types of resources are limited, we do what we can, where we are, with what we have.

And any human with low emotional, financial, time, or knowledge resources may show lower compliance to what would theoretically be expected of him or her than if these resources were available. Thus, burnout, secondary traumatic stress, compassion fatigue, low work engagement, and moral distress come with the territory when we voluntarily overstep outside of our area of expertise in an attempt to provide more for the patients. And the same happens when patients overstep outside of their area of expertise in an attempt to provide more for other patients.

Because some of the healthcare providers and because some of the patients kind of lose themselves in the attempt to save others, in those doing it without sufficient social and psychological support, lassitude has a gradual draining effect. And disturbed sleep is one of the most important causes of humans' non-compliance to literally anything, with most of us being more difficult to deal with and making worse decisions when overly tired (Pearson, 2023).

Many breast cancer patients develop progressively worse sleep during chemotherapy (Savard, 2009). Thereafter, these sleep disturbances are associated with more side effects of treatment and an increased incidence of complications during hospital stays (Vin-Raviv, 2018). Then, frequent nocturnal awakenings, insomnia, or hypersomnia can be further amplified during radiotherapy, with some patients still reporting disturbed sleep even one year after the end of the treatment (Fontes, 2017).

And most put it on the treatment, disregarding the fact that not all individuals with the same treatment develop these disturbances (Costa, 2014).

Moreover, there is a difference between the subjective reports and the objective measurements (Garrett, 2011). A study comparing sleep quality during radiotherapy in breast and prostate cancer patients using the subjective Pittsburgh Sleep Quality Index, the General Sleep Disturbance Scale, the Lee Fatigue Scale, and the objective wrist actigraphy shows that:

- based on self-reports, women experienced sleep disturbance more frequently and with greater severity than men,
- based on objective measures, men were the ones who actually had the more severe sleep disturbances.

So, are distressed women more talkative while essentially preserving better sleep, while men are the ones harder hit by distress and actually having the lower quality sleep but manning up and not talking about it?

The interpersonal differences between different individuals' ability to deal with stress might explain the differences between the self-reported data and the objectively measured ones.

This is important to count as, for instance, irrespective of gender, distinct variations in psychosocial factors such as catastrophizing, anxiety, depression, and distress somatization play an important role in developing persistent pain after breast cancer surgery (Schreiber, 2014). Thus, if sleep disturbances remain unaddressed, they can further amplify patients' non-compliance by the increased experience of chronic pain, hot flashes, or fatigue (Leysen, 2019) and even by an increased discomfort perception associated with lymphedema in a positive feedback loop that gets harder and harder to treat (Bock, 2022).

Sleep is important not only for patients' physical and mental health. Sleep is also important in preserving healthcare providers' capacity for optimal treatment delivery and in preserving their own physical and mental health. For instance, during the COVID-19 pandemic, many healthcare providers reported sleep problems, which amplified their psychological distress (Marvaldi, 2021). I'm mentioning the pandemics as sometimes patients and even those running the healthcare system itself kind of imply that being used to working in stressful conditions somehow makes one better at dealing with stress by default. But despite the expected hormesis:

- About 20% of healthcare providers experienced burnout or post-traumatic stress disorders, especially those younger, female, working frontline, with current or past anxiety or depression, or with low social support (Pappa, 2022).
- Anxiety and depression were significantly higher during the 2nd COVID wave, underlining the need to professionally support healthcare providers' mental health, rest and sleep (Pataka, 2022).

Without any pandemic, shift workers who sleep during the day have higher cortisol levels, which diminishes the healing power of sleep and leads to an average of 1 to 4h of less sleep than those who sleep at night. The resulting sleep debt ends in chronic fatigue, worsening attention, vigilance, cognition, and working memory, thus having a negative impact on work performance and safety (Kayser, 2022); the likelihood of a car crash doubling after one night of < 5h of sleep (Sprajcer, 2023).

Some healthcare providers enjoy the flexibility and financial rewards offered by shift work, but the subsequent increased fatigue, headache or migraines, poor sleep, and more frequent unhealthy behaviors gradually undermine these benefits.

While duty-hour restrictions have been instituted to protect sleep among trainees in the US, for instance, no such effort has been made for attending physicians who have completed their training or for physicians working in nonacademic settings. For these people, there is no policy, process, or training at an organizational, academic, or personal level on how best to manage sleep and fatigue (Kancherla, 2020).

Surgical team burnout is a collective syndrome characterized by a gradually diminished perception of personal accomplishments, emotional exhaustion, depersonalization, and depression caused by the distress encountered throughout their training and career (Meeusen, 2024). When this remains chronically uncompensated by adequate rest, even mild sleep restrictions of 1.5 h/night over six weeks can increase perceived stress and anxiety, especially in those sleeping less than 5h (Benasi, 2024).

For instance, in a study performed on 5579 medical residents in Japan, 15.5% slept less than 5h, and 26.7% had insomnia, thus increasing both the risk of depressive symptoms and the risk of medical errors (Nagasaki, 2024).

Juggling personal and professional life when working night shifts has an impact on nurses too, kind of making the sleep-deprived healthcare providers feel like they are daily living in the Twilight Zone. Working night shifts, high responsibility, long hours, work-family conflict, and insufficient recovery sleep are among the causes of physicians' and nurses' burnout, potentially lowering their ability to provide higher-quality care (Weaver, 2023).

The impact of temporary sleep restrictions can also be hypersensitivity to pain, but these changes can be reversed by day napping (Faraut, 2015). That is, of course, if you nap.

There is no data on the effects of naps on safety outcomes in the workplace, but when possible, data on night-shift napping shows that this short-duration recovery behavior leads to improved performance (Ruggiero, 2014). It is important to brainstorm all possible ways to recover lost sleep, as even in the healthiest of people, insufficient rest accumulated over time increases the risk of:

- anxiety (Cox, 2016),
- depression (Mirchandaney, 2023),
- nonalcoholic fatty liver disease (Yang J. e., 2023),
- diabetes (Cappuccio, 2010), hypertension (Thomas, 2017),
- autoimmune diseases (Hsiao, 2015),
- Alzheimer's disease (Han Z. X., 2024),
- and obesity (Cooper, 2018). Especially abdominal obesity (Sun M. e., 2018).

Of the behavioral pathways linking insufficient sleep with fat gain, eating more and worse quality foods due to deregulated appetite hormones seems the most obvious (Lin J. e., 2020). Nonetheless, insufficient sleep is not only about worsened eating behavior but also about worsened metabolism. RCT data shows that:

- In healthy people:
    - Sleep restrictions reduce insulin sensitivity (Sondrup, 2022).
    - A single night of total sleep deprivation is sufficient to induce anabolic resistance (Lamon, 2021).
    - Performing exercise when sleep-restricted may not provide the same adaptive response for individuals as if they were fully rested (Knowles, 2024).
- In people recently diagnosed with diabetes, for every 30 minutes of daily sleep debt, the fat gain tendency increased by 41% at 12 months (Arora, 2016).

- In overweight or obese people, sleep debt lowers their ability to lose fat even when they purposefully try to. The same diet kept under low sleep conditions leads to weight loss by muscle loss (Nedeltcheva, 2010).

There is no diet or specific food to improve sleep (Netzer, 2024). Thus, to improve it and consequently obtain better personal and professional outcomes, it is important for patients and healthcare providers alike to practice proper sleep hygiene behaviors:

- Try to have consistent sleep patterns, doing your best to respect bedtimes and wake-up times while knowing that when insufficient sleep happens, catch-up sleep is beneficial (Sletten, 2023).
- Adapt the bedroom temperature to your subjective thermal comfort level, considering that indoor temperatures <18°C (Janssen, 2023) and >26°C (Tham, 2020) are currently associated with negative health effects.
- Avoid light exposure during the night (Tähkämö, 2019).
- Limit daytime exposure to blue light from electronic devices, a type of light with a wavelength that influences the circadian rhythm and lowers sleep quality (Silvani, 2022).
- Limit noise exposure (Smith, 2022).
- Spend more time outside during the day, as each additional hour spent outdoors lowers the odds of lifetime major depressive disorder, antidepressant use, anhedonia, neuroticism, and bad mood (Burns, 2021).

However, because, more often than not, disturbed sleep is a manifestation of distress, the most important specialist to address it is a clinical psychologist, although, at times, a psychiatrist might also be needed.

The emotional fatigue part of lassitude can be covered by clinical psychologists, data showing that due to their training, these professionals remain quite balanced when compared with others working in oncology, being able to support themselves, their patients, and their colleagues (Morris, 2021).

Several factors appear to be associated with less burnout in clinical psychologists, including:

- exposure to patients' recovery,
- discussing traumas,
- less moral distress and finding meaning in their work.

Improving self-compassion and reducing self-criticism lead to reduced psychological distress and improved sleep (Norton, 2024). Yet, many people working in oncology experience low compassion even for themselves and talk with no one about their personal distress, although any available support does nothing if you're not using it.

Having access to professional support of any kind has no impact if you're unmotivated to do your part when it comes to at least asking for help.

Third, humans are not robots.

Traditional recommendations for behavior change rely on the assumption that changes occur quickly, dichotomously, and without relapse. However, human behavior is far more complex than this basic assumption, as we don't push a button and change when advised or even when we intentionally choose to (Prochaska, 1991).

The "Just DO it!" motto is not how the human brain works.

It sounds nice; it might work in marketing, and it's how people untrained in behavioral sciences suppose other humans should work. Nevertheless, a real change that needs to be adopted for the long-term is hard for any of us, requiring patience, commitment, and perseverance to successfully go through the six stages of behavioral change:

1. **Precontemplation** – you're unaware that you have an ineffective behavior.
2. **Contemplation** – you become aware that you have one and that you need to change.
3. **Determination** – you look for solutions and kind of try them out.
4. **Action** – you choose the one solution you think fits you and start to apply it frequently with high enthusiasm.
5. **Relapse** – then life slaps you in the face, and you fall back to your familiar routines.
6. **Maintenance** – and then, the people who found solutions to continue to practice the new behavior when the going got rough are the ones who gradually manage to become a healthier version of themselves. Behavioral change is a marathon. Not a sprint.

Swinging like a pendulum between high enthusiastic start, relapse, and give up or kind of restart is the human factor influencing the outcome of all our work, roughly called "non-compliance." But what many do when talking about non-compliance is to refuse their own responsibility for stage-matched personalized interventions while pointing the finger outside themselves (Krebs P. e., 2018), not knowing or choosing to ignore that adhering long-term to a new behavior is deeply emotional:

- People in the Precontemplation stage might not even grasp why we ask them to do certain behaviors, while healthcare professionals with no behavioral sciences training usually have no idea about how to bring resistant

patients to a point where change will ever be seriously contemplated, let alone attempted (Barber, 1994). For instance, some young patients ask if the prognosis is so good, like for a stage I luminal A invasive ductal breast cancer, why on Earth should she take the antiestrogenic medication to make her sexual life hell through vaginal dryness or dyspareunia?!
- The act of understanding the reason behind a potentially beneficial requirement happens in the Contemplation stage, far, far from the real-world Action or Maintenance behaviors. Without having all the therapeutical options explained and the personal values taken into consideration, many young patients diagnosed with good prognosis breast cancers refuse the secondary prevention hell. And because some of the non-compliant patients make progress, but many do not, the refusal of treatment remains a patient right. The only not right part about it is not to communicate their refusal to the healthcare providers.

All stages of change are important for long-term behavioral maintenance, but maybe the most important would be the Determination to start. Or restart. That is because what means the world to me might mean nothing to you, and what's essential to you might seem trivial to me. Without the emotional component of the Determination stage, there is no long-term change, as trying things out does not equal commitment. And emotionally, we choose based on force or power. While force kind of looks like power, the two are diametrically opposite.

Forcing behavioral change by fear, persuasion, coercion, intimidation, or manipulation is not efficient in free-living conditions, even when self-applied. Although many healthcare providers and caregivers think that people diagnosed with cancer should be forced into submission for their own good, a cancer diagnosis doesn't change who patients are as a species.

Forcing change is unproductive in the long-term, even when it comes to health because it insults humans' need for autonomy (Tengland, 2012). Psychological empowerment is a process essential to feeling competent, while stigma associates poor adherence to treatment, mental distress, and an increased risk for recurring health problems (Dolezal, 2022).

Making decisions is emotional; the Determination stage of the behavioral change requires feeling that:

- you personally chose it,
- you are able to do it.

Force doesn't work in free humans. And even if it works in the chained ones, it remains a matter of debate. Of course, there is a thinking process added to the emotional decision as you acknowledge that life may through you a curveball from time to time, but overall, to change long-term, you must feel that this is important enough for you to make an effort and that with your available resources, you are powerful enough to commit.

What humans feel, think, and do is aligned, as we are not rational unless we feel we choose to and that we can be. Being imposed to do something or feeling unable to do it makes people either covertly fake it or overtly refuse to even try. That is why paternalistic medicine doesn't work when the treatment is self-administered by the patient, and that is why empowering patients' self-efficacy and positive decisional balance improves compliance (Toivonen, 2020). If psychological empowerment is missing from the table, so is genuine behavioral change (Barbosa, 2021).

The foundation of behavioral change is a powerful enough "why" to make one find reasons to do something new and potentially frustrating.

And this is the easiest part, as decision-making is highly subjective, being influenced by factors with an emotional impact that is personal to each one of us (LeBlanc, 2015). Furthermore, neurotic, immature, and pathological defense mechanisms are prevalent in the general population, being associated with psychosocial impairment that sometimes gets under the radar (Blanco, 2023).

This can be recognized and professionally addressed by clinical psychologists in the patients or in the healthcare providers willing to both recognize it and ask for help. Thus, the first step for anyone considering a behavioral change is to know where they stand now, as even if we'd like to go from point A to point B, Waze will ask us about the current location.

When it comes to recommending a patient's behavioral change, the assumption that we don't need to know where she stands frequently translates into a short-term covert submissive behavior that gradually becomes obvert non-compliance.

On the one hand, people who currently reside in the drama triangle react to a reasonable request for a changed behavior with fight, flight, or freeze stress reactions. The drama triangle is a theoretical framework proposed in the 1960s by Stephen Karpman. We learn about it in professional nutrition because eating is a behavior. And no behavior changes as long as the focus is on avoiding oneself by attacking, saving, or completely relying on others. Bullies, rescuers, and victims are frequent in oncology settings, but they are not oncology-specific.

Acting like a Victim (damsel in distress), Rescuer (hero), and Persecutor (villain) are self-avoidant behaviors used when perceived psychological empowerment feels low (Lac, 2022), and one looks for ways to defer responsibility and say that the suboptimal outcome is not their fault:

- The fight-stress reaction is an answer to a trigger perceived as more powerful.
- Saving others looks like caring, but how does it help doing your child's homework? Shouldn't she be allowed to make the effort to learn her own life lessons to grow better?
- And sometimes it feels like we're witnessing a misfortune show at a planetary level, as many are whining about who had it worse, who endured more, who had the sadder bad luck.

Self-avoidance by the focus on others is a behavioral strategy used under stress by any people who try to avoid blame or shame by justifying not doing their own part to improve themselves. And nothing grows in the drama triangle except more drama (Karpman, 1968).

There is also the winner's triangle proposed by Acey Choy, an empowering antithesis that eliminates the drama by replacing each of the self-avoidant roles with self-ownership (Choy, 1990). So, from where do humans get the inner power?

The first ingredient of inner power underlined by Acey Choy is owning the responsibility for our behaviors. No one can push another out of the drama triangle until this other human doesn't own their behavior. The emotional reaction to a reasonable request for a changed behavior can be actual change if the person is done with the attacking, saving, or counting on others' drama and if the perceived inner power is high enough to have the required patience, commitment, and resilience.

A behavioral change is not about temporarily acting the part. We actually have to do it consistently.

And while not everything is our fault, we can't do anything about what is not our fault. By taking responsibility, the drama triangle can become the winner's triangle.

Only when we reach the emotional maturity to at least accept that part of the undesired outcome is our fault can we change, as only then do we start to have personal power. No matter how well-intended, potentially beneficial, or scientifically justified, no one can take the pills, no one can do the screening mammography, no one can eat better, no one can improve their sleep, no one can practice physical activity, and no one can learn to communicate better and resolve conflicts instead of yelling, manipulating, shutting down or turning away except for each and every one of us. As Snoop Dogg said in the "I want to thank. Me." speech famous on YouTube, we can only thank ourselves for all our hard work. Or we can continue to blame, save, attack or fully submit to others for the drama we created by avoiding ourselves.

Without ownership, there is no personal power. Without ownership, there is no change. Thus, besides taking ownership, what is inner power made of?

Imagine holding your cortisol-inducing long to-do list in your dominant hand and in your other hand as many dopamine sources as you can possibly afford and also are able to handle. Despite the fact that in the era of consumerism, we're encouraged to just juggle stress with as many supplies of pleasure as we can afford, this is not power. This is forcing yourself through life while using numbing as a band-aid.

"Quality of life" has become such a buzzword nowadays that it has been emptied of the bare heart of it: quality of life largely depends on our decisions.

For instance, eating is a behavior.

Nutrition is a behavioral science. While the metabolic disturbances present in the people under oncology treatments or in the overly tired people administering them can be managed with proper compliance to professional nutrition, these remain on the tables of the people who, for whatever personal reason, made the decision to be a passive recipient either of treatment or of contextual life-work imbalance. When one doesn't do what is told, blame or harsher restrictions only make things worse, gradually amplifying the behavioral disturbances used to numb the distress. And this happens in all behavioral areas.

To make a long story short, inner power is the ability to balance cortisol and dopamine enough to remain moderate under stress, and this is internally built on:

- purpose = vasopressin
- affection = oxytocin
- mood = serotonin
- self-control = γ-Aminobutyric acid (GABA)

Dr. Sue Carter's work on integrative neurobiology shows that the oxytocin-vasopressin pathway is essential to provide a sense of safety and to reduce anxiety or distress (Carter C. S., 1999). Besides keeping themselves down by trying to avoid blame via refusing to take responsibility, people living in the drama triangle are low on one or more of these four internal pillars of inner power, and under stress, they try to compensate for the inner void by binging on any easily available external source of dopamine, in an attempt to somehow cool off the overheated internal engine. There are differences between different people, and there are differences within the same person at different stages of personal development, a cold reality shower being sometimes critical for optimized self-efficacy.

The truth remains, though, that the foundation of humans' inner power is to have both affection and purpose while being in a good mood and having the ability to control themselves.

I started with vasopressin, as humans' responsiveness to the main love hormone is highly dependent on a whole lot of other factors than being shown love, the potential emotional nourishment one might get from the mighty oxytocin being influenced by a myriad of factors:

- bad childhood experiences (Grimm, 2014),
- menstrual cycle-phase (Engel S. e., 2019) or menopause (Maestrini, 2018),
- metabolic homeostasis (Ding C. M.-S., 2019), type 1 (Kujath, 2015) or type 2 diabetes (Qian, 2014),
- social anxiety (Tabak, 2022), and
- burnout (Simpkin, 2020).

Paradoxically, stress-deregulated sensitivity to oxytocin can also be manifested as increased fear, avoidance, and antisocial behavior. This reinforces the importance of considering context and personal factors when evaluating the impact of perceived affection on behavior (Szymanska, 2017). Even previous pet exposure matters when it comes to being able to perceive the love expressed by a pet. The higher the stress, the lower the response to the oxytocin ability to make us feel loved and the lower the capacity to trust ourselves or others (Curry, 2015). Simply owning a dog, for instance, doesn't necessarily lead to more oxytocin. To achieve the beneficial impact of affection, the desirable dog-owner interaction resulting in increased oxytocin levels and decreased cortisol depends on the way the owners interact with their dogs (Petersson, 2017).

Passivity doesn't work when it comes to affection.

While many healthcare providers untrained in behavioral sciences are only aware of vasopressin's impact on cardiovascular and renal homeostasis, the antidiuretic hormone is actually a multitasking peptide that also regulates social behaviors involved in cooperation, competition, isolation, and loneliness (Glavaš, 2022).

Because of the detrimental impact stress has on responsivity to oxytocin, and because the chemical structure of vasopressin is similar to the one of oxytocin, vasopressin can bond to oxytocin receptors when oxytocin is low, potentially being the main bonding hormone used by those living chronically burdened with risks and stress (Kareklas, 2024). Through the positive emotions they still manage to feel when problem-solving with others, distressed people may be more internally driven to use work and sports performance as a way to bond (Brunnlieb, 2016).

Moreover, vasopressin may be the most important neuroendocrine basis for men's personal power to maintain work and physical performance and to avoid fear and anxiety (Litvin, 2013).

Preclinical data shows that testosterone and its metabolites influence social recognition in males primarily through the Vasopressin 1a receptor (Gabor, 2012), while human data shows that men who internally feel more competent have higher vasopressin levels which are related to a larger social network, fewer negative marital interactions, and more secure attachment (Gouin, 2012). But while vasopressin can get things going by providing the practicality of things, complex behavioral functions, including affectionate, sexual behaviors, social bonds, and parenting, are not just about going through the motion as they require the combined activity of both vasopressin and oxytocin (Carter C. S., 2017).

One vital gift from vasopressin is that it makes things fun and exciting, making the difference between peace and boredom. Actually, doing things together with our loved ones makes us bond. And we're kind of witnessing a dual epidemic of disturbed oxytocin and vasopressin, as in the social media age, people gradually started to rely on all sorts of virtual friendships to replace the time spent together in real life. But contrary to the modern swipe-left era, humans remain social creatures.

We need a true emotional connection with each other to internally function well. And since cortisol blocks oxytocin receptors, what most people tend to do under stress is to go to work. Or maybe to the gym, as in the case of people who also get a drive out of physical performance. But more and more people are sedentary and, over the years, the need to contribute to society through meaningful work has gotten lower and lower in the younger generations, frequently dismissed as the low motivation of millennials.

When things start to go sideways, even at work, what we get when both oxytocin and vasopressin are low is withdrawal, social isolation, and a feeling of boredom and loneliness, even inside the family unit. These are consequences of the reduced ability or interest to do one's part when the perceived affection reward is low (Crespi, 2022), being related to poor physical and mental health, substance use, stigma, and constant perception of ill-treatment by others while you're absent yourself (Ingram, 2020).

Without the purpose and fun brought in by work and/or sports, and without the emotional reward of loving relationships, all one's got is boredom and loneliness, falling easy prey to the highs and lows of cortisol and dopamine addictive pathways.

The serotonin-improved mood is another pillar of internal power, being able to stimulate the release of vasopressin and oxytocin when the going gets rough (Jørgensen, 2003).

Unlike in the case of vasopressin, more healthcare providers are aware of serotonin's impact on moods and behaviors due to its mainstream association with depression (Moncrieff, 2023). However, things go deeper than that, as there are well-established roles of serotonin in cardiovascular and gastrointestinal physiology (Jonnakuty, 2008), while newer data shows its importance in bone health (Lavoie, 2017) and in preventing obesity by maintaining proper insulin secretion and glycemic control (Georgescu, 2021).

The problem with getting to the internal peace offered by serotonin is that about 90% is secreted in the cells lining our gastrointestinal tract, and only about 10% is produced in the brain. When all is well with our intestines, serotonin promotes prosocial behaviors through internal calm. However, all diagnoses, treatments, and eating behaviors affecting the intestinal mucosal integrity can diminish the ability to maintain calm under stress by lowering the intestinal secretion of serotonin (Stasi, 2019).

Inner peace turns to outer war by dysbiosis-associated serotonin deficiency. Inflammatory bowel disease (González Delgado, 2022), antibiotics (Ge X. e., 2017), chemotherapy (Bajic, 2018), alcohol (Chen G. e., 2022), artificial sweeteners (Chae, 2024), or the nowadays so popular weight loss GLP-1 receptor agonist treatments like semaglutide that may associate delayed gastric emptying (Wei L. e., 2021), and pretty much all other things with intestinal side effects are able to disturb the serotoninergic system.

And casually throwing all sorts of supplements or supportive medications with intestinal side effects on top of the curative oncology treatments instead of referring the patient to true supportive care obtainable by professional nutrition may amplify both the disturbed mood and the drug-induced nutritional disorders (Yalçın, 2019).

Furthermore, the fact that the same intestines responsible for the serotonin-induced inner peace are the human body part also responsible for the best part of non-specific immunity, and the fact that serotonin is released into our bloodstream and absorbed by platelets, build together the anatomical basis of the psycho-immunity bridge between mental, immunological, and coagulation-related disorders (Izzi, 2020).

Interventions using dietary depletion of the serotonin precursor tryptophan show that serotonin-depleted people are more likely to punish those who treat them unfairly and slower to accept fair exchanges, with serotonin deficiency increasing the tendencies of hypervigilance and vengeance (Crockett, 2013). When the serotoninergic system is dysregulated, what we get instead of inner peace is righteousness.

The ability to tell ourselves no is offered by GABA, the last pillar of personal power being the main inhibitory neurotransmitter in the brain. It has anatomic and functional connectivity both with oxytocin and dopamine, correlating low perceived affection with:

- substance use addictions like alcohol use disorder (Wang Z. e., 2022) or binge eating (Novelle M. G., 2018),
- non-substance use addictions like smartphone addiction (Seo, 2020) or gambling disorder (Møller, 2019).

When we're not aware of what's causing the distress and only focus on the effect of the distress, those things causing distress will continue to cause distress, amplifying the neurosis manifested as the many coping behaviors. And as Carl Yung said, "We do not cure neurosis; neurosis cures us." Thus, these many coping behaviors under stress may be part of the attempt to self-care.

There is an ongoing debate about the food addiction concept, as many behavioral scientists, psychologists, and neuroscientists tend to agree more on the addiction to the act of eating itself than on the addiction to specific foods (Wilcox, 2021). When it comes to binge eating, compulsive grazing, or emotional eating, most approve that patients with any of these eating addictive behaviors display similar symptoms to those experienced by drug addicts, having deregulated responses to dopamine, oxytocin, serotonin, and GABA (Novelle M. G., 2021).

People who don't have enough meaning in their lives are more prone to addiction, as when vasopressin, oxytocin, serotonin, and GABA are not there to save the day during a stressful day, a dopamine rush can seem like heaven.

If one is unaware of the neurochemistry of inner power, one only sees the displayed behavioral consequence. To better picture this, let's consider the fact that the dysbiosis associated with serotonin and GABA deficiency is frequent in people with chronic pain (Garvey, 2023). So, after breast cancer surgery, how much of the reported chronic pain is surgical treatment-related, and how much is dysbiosis-related?

When people feel temporarily better on the short bursts obtained from binging on dopamine, we see some short-lived compliance. Hooray! But then, when the numbing runs off, they slide back to craving dopamine due to the disrupted vasopressin, oxytocin, serotonin, and GABA. This is what makes it hard to maintain a behavior that you rationally know is good for you. While some might see the short-lived compliance as better than nothing, inconsistency fuels addiction as the unresolved distress temporarily glazed over by the dopamine binge gradually increases the need for even more numbing (Rassool, 2011). Addiction is the most detrimental part of living internally drained under unpredictable and intermittent access to potential pleasurable triggers (Clark, 2023).

And there's nothing wrong with dopamine; we all enjoy it. But to enjoy it instead of numbing with it, it has to be kind of like fireworks: shining in the dark but also rare and brief.

How much would we still enjoy fireworks if it would last for two hours, scheduled every Thursday, during lunch?

Consistent proper behavior requires adequate responsiveness to oxytocin, the inner calm associated with serotonin, the congruence offered by GABA's gift of the ability to self-restrain, and the consideration of other people accessible through vasopressin.

All these four pillars are the neurobiological foundation of the internal ability to trust. Ourselves or others.

When surviving with an inner void with a chronic cortisol/dopamine ± vasopressin war mode on, this can be any of us. And blaming oneself or others for not doing a "should" puts gas on the fire, as the need to use addiction to self-soothe is amplified by shame (Snoek, 2021).

If we put the focus on the people diagnosed with cancer, many see-saw between cortisol and dopamine as, at least temporarily, they lose the vasopressin as they can no longer work and feel like other performance-related activities are not a priority when they fight for their life, sometimes they lose oxytocin as they divorce or have relationship issues with their partners, sometimes they lose their ability to self-restrain or start to adopt defeatism by taking to extremes otherwise healthy behaviors, or they find no way to self-sooth the many physical and emotional side effects of oncology treatments.

If we put the focus on the people working with those diagnosed with cancer, many hang on vasopressin for dear life, forcing themselves with all their might to do more and more meaningful work while also see-sawing between cortisol and dopamine as sometimes they lose oxytocin as they divorce or have relationship issues with their partners, sometimes they lose their ability to self-restraint or start to adopt defeatism by taking to extremes otherwise healthy behaviors, or they find no way to self-soothe the many physical and emotional side effects of administering oncology treatments.

And yes, I wrote the almost same sentence twice as we are incredibly alike.

For anyone working or being treated in oncology settings while living in the drama triangle jail due to the inner emptiness generated by low vasopressin, oxytocin, serotonin, or GABA, it takes highly trained psychotherapists to show the inmates shaking the prison bars for dear life that the door is wide open.

It's called "non-compliance," but it's about drained humans with low trust.

Is it a ridiculous idea to drop the double standard?

Chapter 6
Alcohol intake

Because most people have zero training in behavioral sciences and most of those in need of behavioral change go to work and then to the fridge or to the bar to obtain some relief under stress, "To drink or not to drink?" remains the question although many casual drinkers, healthcare professionals or not, seem unaware that alcohol carcinogenity is a fact.

The causal link between excessive alcohol intake and cancer is somewhat accepted, although many do not acknowledge it in their day-to-day life, the risk looking higher for spirits than for other drinks (Petri, 2004). However, it seems that light and moderate alcohol intake can also be carcinogenic, with statistics estimating that 4.1% of breast cancers are attributable to light intake, defined as exceeding one drink per month (Mostofsky, 2024).

And for those ignoring the predictable irrationality of emotionally depleted humans under stress, data published during the COVID pandemic shows that essential workers like healthcare providers who used to just drink a beer in a pub after work before the pandemic then drunk the whole bottle of wine at home instead (Sallie, 2020). Consequently, 741300 of the new cancer cases diagnosed in the first year of COVID-19 were attributable to alcohol consumption, among which esophagus, liver, colorectal, and breast cancers (Rumgay, 2021).

Acetaldehyde—the toxic metabolite of alcohol that is used to cause cancer in laboratory animals—might explain the associations between cancer and light-to-moderate intake. The higher its intake, the higher the amount of reactive oxygen species that can damage DNA, thus increasing the carcinogenic effect (Seitz, 2012). Nevertheless, cancer-specific mortality risk associated with light and moderate alcohol consumption remains somewhat in the eye of the beholder:

- When sick people, former alcoholics, and never drinkers are all classified as "non-drinkers," we get a systematic overestimation error (Naimi, 2017), "moderate drinkers" having lower cancer-specific mortality when compared with "non-drinkers" and with "any current drinkers"—which is the famous J-shaped French Paradox (Tjønneland, 2007).
- When "lifetime abstinent" people are compared with "any current drinkers," what we get is a dose-dependent positive association with cancer-specific mortality, even for light intake (Ko H. e., 2021).

Epidemiological studies are not proof of causality, but they are easier to do, publish and endorse.

Epidemiological studies' conclusions related to alcohol may be biased by obesity, menopausal status (Fagherazzi, 2015), smoking (Cao Y. e., 2015), and sedentary work (Lee J. e., 2021). The general trend is that the personal ability to sustain an overall healthy lifestyle is paramount for breast cancer primary or secondary prevention, the risk increasing when moderation flies out the window, even with rare binge drinking episodes defined as consuming more than five drinks per day (Chen W. Y., 2011).

Epidemiological alcohol data is a cocktail of results based on the following:

- **Study design:** different researchers use different definitions for "non-drinker," the bad health of former alcoholics, and of sick people who stopped drinking for medical reasons, being part of the evidence behind the moderate alcohol intake benefits (Fillmore, 2006).
- **Recall bias:** most of the available studies are based on self-reported questionnaire data.
- **Unadjusted data for immunohistochemistry and ethnicity.**

When "non-drinkers" include only "never drinkers," the available breast cancer-specific data separated by histology and immunohistochemistry shows:

- a twofold increased risk of HR+ invasive lobular, luminal A breast cancers (Li C. I., 2010),
- a slight association with the HER2 positive breast cancers (Hirko, 2016), and
- no association with triple-negative breast cancers (Kumar N. e., 2024), except among Black women (Young, 2023).

Nonetheless, despite genetic differences influencing alcohol impact on women of different ethnicities, the broad lack of association with triple-negative breast cancers is taken one step further by the Metropolitan Detroit and Los Angeles County SEER registry data, astonishingly concluding that the younger the age at alcohol use initiation associates the lower the risk of triple-negative young-onset breast cancer (Hirko, 2024). Subsequent marketing messages promoting alcohol intake as part of a breast cancer-preventing healthy lifestyle are part of the pinkwashing corporate campaigns in which the sponsoring company positions itself as a fighter against breast cancer while promoting products and behaviors that increase breast cancer risk (Mart, 2015).

And what the public gets from data implying that younger age at alcohol intake initiation is protective against the harsh triple-negative breast cancers, and from the pinkwashing campaigns promoting alcohol as a part of a healthy lifestyle meant to prevent cancer, is outright confusion and a reason to keep on unhealthy behaviors for those who wish to keep them. Consequently, current drinking is common among the US cancer survivors, with many exceeding moderate intake even while on active cancer treatment:

- 77.7% of young survivors drink alcohol regularly,
- 23.8% meet the criteria for binge drinking (Shi, 2023).

Breast cancer-specific mortality seems to go down with one drink per month in some studies (Flatt S. W., 2010) and up with two drinks per day in others (Gou, 2013). The correlation with a higher recurrence risk in patients who continue to drink after the diagnosis vs. in those who stop drinking is reported especially in postmenopausal and overweight or obese women (Simapivapan, 2016)—"yet, the cardioprotective effect of alcohol on non-breast cancer death is suggested" (Kwan, 2010) despite the higher all-cause mortality associated even with low alcohol intake (Zhao J. e., 2023).

There are many contradicting messages about alcohol. We have VIP breast cancer survivors promoting wine intake on mainstream media, while the Earth is looking in dismay at how the French have their buttery delicious pastry and eat it too…

The carcinogenic and the cardioprotective impacts of alcohol bud heads even in researchers, maybe because the 200+ year-old cardioprotective story of alcohol is quite older than the 30+ year-old acknowledgment that alcohol is a carcinogen.

In the *Clinical and Pathological Reports* by Samuel Black, published in 1819, the Irish doctor wrote that angina pectoris is much less common in France than in Ireland. That's pretty much all there is to is the 200+ year-old cardioprotective story of alcohol. Ever since, epidemiological study after study has gradually created the subliminal message that light-to-moderate alcohol consumption is important for preventing cardiovascular disease (Ronksley, 2011), although even cardiologists acknowledge that the available scientific literature shows nothing except correlations (Goel, 2018).

Some studies suggest that red wine is beneficial (Serio, 2023). Others suggest that wine of any color confers cardiovascular protection (Lucerón-Lucas-Torres, 2023). Others conclude that wine and beer confer greater cardiovascular protection than spirits based on their non-alcoholic components—mainly polyphenols (De Gaetano, 2016). At the same time, others imply that ethanol in any alcoholic drink brings cardiovascular benefits (Krnic, 2011). The role of wine in explaining the French paradox is questionable, as its' unique effects on longevity may be indirectly biased by the lower socioeconomic status of non-wine drinkers—people with lower financial means, smoking more, being more sedentary, and having an overall inferior health (Holahan, 2012). Still, the lower socioeconomic status of non-wine drinkers is typically ignored.

The oldest hypothesis is that moderate alcohol intake prevents atherosclerosis by inhibiting atheromatosis via increased blood levels of high-density lipoproteins cholesterol (HDL-c) and decreased low-density lipoproteins cholesterol (LDL-c). How this happens is neither fully understood nor proven.

- Some researchers suggest that alcohol increases HDL-c by increasing the transport rate of apolipoprotein A1 (De Oliveira e Silva, 2000).

- Others report that long-term alcohol consumption, even in small amounts, causes a significant decrease in HDL-c by decreasing the transport rate of apolipoprotein A1 (Cho, 2022).
- Others explained the cardioprotective story by alcohol stimulating cells' cholesterol efflux and its esterification in plasma (Sierksma, 2004).
- Others report it based on a 3.45 to 3.34 LDL-c decrease (Baer, 2002).

While 0.09 is mathematically bigger than 0, cholesterol level is multifactorial, involving smoking, stress, physical exercise, food eaten, BMI, age, sex, and genetic factors (Nindita, 2023). Singling out drinking from all of these does not render the others irrelevant. Data shows that people with lower HDL-c levels are more likely to have low incomes, an unhealthy lifestyle, and other comorbidities (Ko D. T., 2016). Even neighborhood unemployment may lead to poor health among all people living there, independent of their own employment status (Hammarström, 2024). So, would a poor person improve cardiovascular health by starting to drink as a health-inducing behavior?

Another hypothesis promotes moderate alcohol intake for stroke prevention based on its antithrombotic effects. In healthy people with no cardiovascular risk factor, randomized trial data reports improved endothelial function and reduced von Willebrand factor only for 30 g of alcohol intake from wine of any color and from beer (Tousoulis, 2008). However, this potential benefit would come from an amount three times higher than the assumed moderate 10 g a day (Stote, 2016).

In breast cancer settings, if moderate alcohol intake would be cardioprotective, it would be only logical to recommend it to patients under trastuzumab or chemotherapy—which are the main breast cancer treatments with cardiac side effects.

The maximal cardiovascular disease protection is reported to be 33%, obtained at 25 g of alcohol intake per day (Costanzo, 2011). However, we have a published study that shows that—contradictory to the epidemiological assumption—breast cancer patients who consumed 25 g/day of alcohol per day during trastuzumab treatment have higher cardiac toxicity (Lemieux, 2013).

Cardioprotection of moderate alcohol intake doesn't seem to occur in people with hypertension (Fuchs, 2021). Irrespective of the HDL-c/LDL-c data, alcohol intake increases de novo synthesis of triglycerides; hypertriglyceridemia is an independent cardiovascular risk factor (Tenenbaum, 2014).

Moreover, the genetic differences influencing alcohol impact are there even when related to cardiovascular health, as Asian populations have an increased risk of hypertension, ischemic and hemorrhagic stroke at the same moderate alcohol intake when compared to non-Asian populations (Millwood, 2019). Immediately after and up to 24h, any alcohol consumption consumed by any human is associated with higher acute cardiovascular risk (Mostofsky, 2016).

And leaving hypotheses aside, alcohol intake influences human health in more ways than one.

Ethanol is absorbed mainly in the stomach and in the small intestine, having a cumulative negative impact on gram-negative commensal bacteria (Patel S. e., 2015). Moderate but regular alcohol intake promotes dysbiosis and leaky gut syndrome, the deregulated microbiome contributing to the pathogenesis of cardiovascular (Lau K. e., 2017) and to a gradual loss of inner peace by diminished ability to secrete serotonin (Chen G. e., 2022).

Ethanol's detrimental impact doesn't stop here. More of these bacteria's lipopolysaccharides are transported to the liver through the portal vein, where they are recognized by Kupffer cells as antigens, leading to cytokine release. And while that was a mouthful of science that maybe you're not in the mood for, please bear with me for a little bit longer. This cytokine release recruits macrophages and neutrophils into the area, promoting a hepatic inflammatory response that progressively leads to liver disease (Fairfield, 2021). This mechanism happens in anyone with chronic alcohol consumption (Mendes, 2020), but it is amplified in people with nonalcoholic fatty liver disease (Seitz, 2015). Paradoxically, the association of light-to-moderate alcohol intake with fatty liver disease is stronger for people with normal weight (Chang, 2020). At hepatic level:

- **Alcohol is first transformed into acetaldehyde:**
  o mainly catalyzed by alcohol-dehydrogenase – with NAD^+ to NADH + H^+ cofactor
- **Acetaldehyde is then transformed into acetate:**
  o catalyzed by acetaldehyde-dehydrogenase – with NAD^+ to NADH + H^+ cofactor.

The more ethanol is consumed, the more NADH is produced. And because NADH stimulates lipogenesis and inhibits lipolysis, any level of alcohol intake is harmful to the liver (Jarvis, 2022). I will write the last part one more time, as regardless of professional training, many people either refuse to acknowledge this to keep their cortisol/dopamine binge on the table or don't grasp it: after a meal where alcohol was consumed, lipogenesis is stimulated, and lipolysis stops.

Many healthcare providers encourage their patients to have a moderate alcohol intake from time to time in order to lower cardiovascular disease risk stepping outside their professional expertise, by casually playing "nutritionist".

But even if this would not be built on data biased by the many subjective work definitions of "current drinkers" and "moderate intake," the single focus on the implied positive cardiovascular effects ignores that, in reality, anything has both positives and negatives and that we need to acknowledge alcohol's negative side effects:

- the carcinogenic impact,
- the dysbiosis-induced serotonin deficiency and cardiovascular toxicity, and
- the hepatic toxicity.

Nevertheless, the "one drink a day" is more popular than the "5 a day" recommended fruit and vegetable intake. Thus, what is "one drink"?

As in the case of the "non-drinkers" definition, the "one standard drink" definition is also fluid, with different countries having different governmental definitions pretty much based on culture, regional tolerance for alcohol and preferences (WHO, 2018). "One standard drink" contains:

- 8 g of pure alcohol in the UK,
- 10 in Australia, Israel, France, and the Netherlands,
- 12 in Sweden and Italy,
- 14 in the US,
- 15 in Chile and Germany,
- 16 in Czechia, and
- 20 in Austria.[4]

There are even countries like Switzerland where the government hasn't yet decided whether one standard drink is 10 or 12 grams. And then there's Norway, which also officially varies but between 12 and 14. Besides the fact that we pretty

---

[4] https://apps.who.int/gho/data/view.main.56470

much don't know whose standard drink is a standard drink, the behavioral pattern called "moderate intake" also varies widely from country to country, ranging for women from 10 to 42 grams per day (Kalinowski, 2016).

The fact that most epidemiological data on alcohol is self-reported means that the studies' results may vary by individual awareness of what a drink is vs. what a drink is arbitrarily decided to be by different authorities. Many people have no clue what one standard drink is in their country or anywhere else, reporting drinking or not drinking "moderately" based on the number of glasses. Hence, studies from different countries may define higher alcohol intakes as "moderate" by governmental definition, and studies built on self-reported data may define higher alcohol intakes as "moderate" by personal definition.

We can joke about how carrots improve vision while alcohol doubles it. And this is not about telling healthy people to stop enjoying their glass of wine in the evening.

Most people who drink will continue to do so, as decisions are mainly based on emotions and only thereafter justified with anything one might see as the reason for the already chosen behavior. Nevertheless, according to the current scientific literature, there is no reason for an abstainer to start drinking, as the level of alcohol consumption that improves health is zero standard drinks per week (Griswold, 2018). People who are able to keep their drinking in moderation are able to be moderate in other areas of their lives, the adjustment for an overall healthier lifestyle wiping out any implied cardioprotection (Biddinger, 2022). Thus, if there is something healthy about moderate alcohol intake, it is the ability to be moderate.

Chapter 7
Smoking

Back in the heat of the COVID pandemic, I remember reading the French study about smoking lowering its incidence and being transported pretty much like Marcel Proust back in time to his aunt Léonie's kitchen by the smell of madeleines, back in time to Boston in 2018 by the smell of absurdity. I was at a sponsored workshop at the American Society for Nutrition conference. Feeling cold (because in American buildings, the air conditioning is set at only 16 degrees, which feels like Alaska for most Europeans) and hungry (because the main things easily available to consume at many of these conferences are fast food and American coffee, which feels like rainwater for most Europeans), I watched in amazement how three top professors tried to prove that soft drinks are healthier than water. The truth be told, only the first two did the job, bringing seemingly scientific arguments to prove that cola is better for humans than water. I still wonder in dismay today: To God damn whom?! The third one, a bit more Tarzan, broke down their pseudo-scientific arguments one by one. Helen Fisher would have probably commented on me feeling a rush of oxytocin, to feeling cold and hungry. But, well, I'm a geek :)

I still remember the organizers standing on the sidelines of the room. Their facial color changed from pink bonbon, delighted by the first two presentations, to brown cola during the third. The faces of the first two presenters also turned brown cola during the third presentation, but what the hell were they thinking? Theoretically, any person with or without a PhD in nutritional sciences would be shocked to attend a nutrition workshop held at the king's party designed to prove that you become healthier if you drink cola rather than if you drink water.

Even the intake of the promoted "healthier" artificially sweetened soda drinks is associated with a higher risk of obesity, type 2 diabetes, hypertension, cardiovascular disease incidence, and higher all-cause mortality (Diaz, "Artificially sweetened beverages and health outcomes: an umbrella review.", 2023). Conflicts of interest bias the available data on the benefits of consuming artificially sweetened beverages effects, even when related to weight control (Mandrioli, 2016), exactly as in the case of e-cigarettes promoted as a "healthier" way to smoke (Kennedy, 2019). The fact that you are a top professor saying inanities does not change the inanities. It only changes your image as an impartial expert by putting a label on your forehead saying that you're for sale.

I relived the same astonishment while reading the Sorbonne Université study concluding that "daily smokers have a significantly lower probability of developing a symptomatic or severe SARS-CoV-2 infection as compared to the general population," just as I was shocked in Boston by the lovely lectures meant to prove that cola protects humans' metabolism.

This was basically a statistical analysis that calculated the incidence of coronavirus infection compared between those who self-reported smoking and those who just said they didn't smoke (Miyara, 2020).

And the French were not the only ones observing humans from the helicopter and concluding we were all blondes. The same unexpectedly low prevalence of smokers among hospitalized COVID-19 patients was reported at the time by an Italian multicenter case-control study published in the Nicotine and Tobacco Research journal (Meini, 2021).

Witnessing first-hand how scientists can be farmed to prove that soda beverages improve health at one of the largest international nutrition conferences felt as stupefying as reading about the benefits of smoking during a pandemic of infectious respiratory disease. Common sense was not that common in those days.

From the herd immunity proposed by the English boss to the disinfectant injections proposed by the American boss to the casual sex as a method of maintaining mental health proposed by the Danish boss, somehow, it also had to come down to smoking. At the moment, they were a little busy dealing with all the pandemic stuff to have the time to investigate whether the metabolic beneficial effects of cola could also protect against COVID-19.

Despite the circus, a review of 26 observational studies and eight meta-analyses was conducted on the 12th of May 2020 on smoking and COVID-19 by the WHO, underlining the poor data quality of hospital-based studies that correlated self-reported patient characteristics with complex health outcomes and concluding that smoking is associated with increased severity of disease and higher mortality in hospitalized COVID-19 patients (WHO, 2020).

The studies that assess the real impact of smoking on human health don't just consider a self-reported "yes" or "no" answer as evidence for the smoking status of a person. This is objectively confirmed by blood and urine tests showing whether a person smokes.

Obviously, these studies are more difficult to do, and during the pandemic, there was no time for such minute details, so the people surveyed in the French, Italian, and many Chinese observational studies were not tested in any way to assess whether the self-reported answer about their smoking was real or not. But without objectively verifying a subjective answer, people can respond to whatever they consider appropriate to get by in the moment.

Self-reported smoking abstinence has been a longtime issue in hospitalized patients; for instance, an older study performed on 9740 Scottish men and women aged 40–59 years old shows that those with a diagnosis of coronary heart disease reported that they had tried to reduce their cigarette consumption or had quit much more often than what was shown objectively by their biochemical measurement of tobacco smoke inhalation assessment by cotinine. Under-reporting was even more prevalent in women than men (Woodward, 1992). Another older study also showed that hospitalized patients with cardiac and respiratory disease were much more likely to lie about their smoking than those with other diseases as they were often acutely aware that their smoking might have contributed to their illness and thus worry about blame, disapproval, and inadequate treatment (Bittoun, 1991).

And one can answer exactly how panic dictates when asked whether you smoke or not amid a worldwide pandemic of respiratory disease. With the lockdown, the widespread fear, and no cure in sight, most of humanity was in high distress back then. If you said you didn't smoke, you didn't risk anyone blaming you for taking up the coronavirus infection, and you didn't risk not being treated well because how the heck would you still smoke when you were repeatedly warned not to touch your mouth with your hands until after you washed them 15 times. Even if you smoked ever since you were 16, now you can remain calm. You were officially a non-smoker, and you got to be treated like any other human because getting infected was not your fault.

Additionally, people may self-report what they actually label as smoking, and many of the people vaping e-cigarettes consider them a risk-free alternative to classic cigarette smoking (Mravec, 2020). To not even mention Sweden, the European country with the lowest smoking rate, where 36% of 9th graders have a daily intake of tobacco as snus (Raninen, 2023), or the many women putting their babies at risk by using snus during pregnancy (Brinchmann, 2023).

Chewing tobacco is a habit in South Asia too, potentially leading to infertility, pregnancy complications, and adverse fetal outcomes, including low birth weight and preterm birth (Itumalla, 2024). But while oral intake of tobacco kind of gets under the radar, more than 50 years of research show a detrimental health impact even for second-hand smoking.[5]

Thus are we talking about tobacco intake, or are we blurring the lines by talking about smoke?

Globally, over 1 billion people are officially "smokers" (Dai, 2022), and maybe during the days of the pandemic, it was a good idea to calm them down by keeping aside that:

- Smoking increases the incidence of infectious diseases and worsens prognosis in a dose-dependent manner (Jiang C. Q., 2020).
- Smoking e-cigarettes is an independent risk factor for respiratory diseases (Bhatta, 2020).
- Smokers with respiratory infections have an increased risk of developing more severe diseases that would require hospital and ICU admission (Han L. e., 2019).

---

[5] https://stacks.cdc.gov/view/cdc/77893

- Smoking increases the risk of diseases associated with a severe COVID-19 evolution or death:
  - Smoking increases the risk of cardiovascular disease (Gallucci, 2020), including:
    - non-smokers exposed to second-hand smoke (Khoramdad, 2020),
    - smokers of e-cigarettes (Espinoza-Derout, 2022),
    - those consuming flavored tobacco by water pipe/hookah smoking (Bhatnagar, 2019),
    - those using snus (Gupta, 2018).
  - Smoking increases the risk of chronic kidney disease in direct proportion to the number of cigarettes smoked per day and the number of years you've been smoking (Xia, 2017).
  - Smoking increases the risk of diabetes even in passive non-smokers exposed to second-hand smoke (Qin G.-Q. e., 2023).
- Smoking increases the risk of chronic obstructive pulmonary disease, and once hospitalized, smokers with COPD have an increased risk of COVID-19 mortality (Zhao Q. e., 2020). Nonetheless, the pandemic is over. Let's get back to oncology.

Smoking cessation is an essential cancer prevention strategy, as deaths due to cancers caused by tobacco increased globally from 1.5 million in 1990 to 2.5 million in 2019 (Sharma, 2023). But some argue that we're more than 7 billion people on the planet and that we're all going to die anyway, so we might as well choose something fun. Just that cancer ain't no fun, and even passive exposure to smoke significantly increases the risk of lung cancer for non-smokers (Jayes, 2016).

Nevertheless, many smokers keep on reminding others that only 15% of all smokers get lung cancers and that not all people with lung cancers are smokers (Kuśnierczyk, 2023). Thus, why stop?!

This is an old discussion, as data going all the way back to the late '50s shows that even then, scientists pleaded for smoking cessation based on the causal link between smoking and lung cancer (Cornfield, 1959). There is more than one type of lung cancer, and the evidence is looking stronger for the small and squamous cell subtypes.

Of course, no single cause accounts for all lung cancers, but the causal link is there, and it has been there for a long time (Lee P. N., 2012). And is there also for the stomach (Rota, 2024), bladder (Jubber, 2023), and pancreatic cancer (Weissman, 2020). While these are mainly researched with regard to tobacco smoking, maybe the worst type of cancer related to smokeless tobacco is head and neck cancer, with patients requiring intensive treatments that are often disfiguring and debilitating for life (Pedroso, 2023). Thus, when talking about smoking carcinogenity, maybe we need to keep in mind that we're talking about tobacco regardless of the intake pathway and that the low number of smokers who actually get lung cancer does not wipe out the other cancers caused by tobacco.

Smoking is not scientifically proven to cause primary breast cancer risk, as although some relative risk is there, the numbers are low, ranging from 1.07 for current smokers to 1.09 for ever smokers (Scala, 2023). However, continuing to smoke after a breast cancer diagnosis is correlated with a 28% increase in breast cancer-specific mortality (Sollie, 2017). Moreover, patients with breast cancer who continue to both drink and smoke after the diagnosis have increased contralateral breast cancer risk (Knight, 2017). These may happen for more than one reason.

Smoking during breast cancer chemotherapy does not influence treatment efficacy (Simon, 2020). But there is more to breast cancer treatment than pCR, and people don't only die of breast cancer.

Cardiotoxicity is the main issue when it comes to smoking during systemic treatment, and while many try to cure cancer without killing the heart, they don't always acknowledge or inform the patient of her part in taking care of her heart during the oncology treatments (Kirkham, 2019). Depending on her inner power and life circumstances, she may choose to do something about it, or she may not, but in day-to-day oncology practice, many are not aware that this is an issue enough to consistently make referrals for smoking cessation professionals (Nolan, 2019).

Because harsher systemic treatments like anthracycline chemotherapy and anti-HER2 targeted treatments are associated with cardiovascular side effects, and because smoking in itself has cardiovascular side effects, it is mainly recognized that combining the two may amplify the treatment-related cardiotoxicity by the patient-related risk factor (Mehta, 2018). However, smoking increased cardiotoxicity may also happen for the newer drugs like elacestrant, tucatinib, neratinib, olaparib, pembrolizumab, or sacituzumab govitecan (Zagami, 2024). This may also happen if smoking continues during the oral administration of the less aggressive capecitabine (Polk, 2016), aromatase inhibitors (Khosrow-Khavar, 2020) or CDK 4/6 inhibitors (Pavlovic, 2023).

And while smoking may also increase the risk of drug-induced interstitial lung disease in patients with breast cancer under treatments like trastuzumab deruxtecan (Rugo, 2023), the take-home message remains that the patient is not a passive recipient of treatment, as the reported treatment-related toxicity is not only treatment-related.

While careful patient selection is recommended and usually performed in oncology, sometimes patient-related behaviors like smoking are not taken into consideration to personalize treatment.

The absolute risks of modern radiotherapy may outweigh the benefits in smokers because continuing to smoke during this breast cancer treatment stage may:

- diminish the net effect radiotherapy has on mortality (Taylor C. e., 2017),
- increase the risks of dermatitis, especially if obesity and smoking collide (Xie, 2021),
- increase cardiac and lung toxicity (Wong G. e., 2020), and
- increase the risk of second primary cancer occurrence (DiMarzio, 2018).

Smoking is also an independent risk factor for many types of early and late postoperative complications after breast reconstructive surgery, the risk multiplying when this behavior is practiced by obese patients previously treated with radiotherapy (Thorarinsson, 2017). Smoking is also a significant risk factor for wound complications following reduction mammaplasty (Hillam, 2017). While there is no ideal breast reconstruction suitable for all patients, former smokers have twice the risk for donor site complications, which remains among the main concerns when it comes to patients accepting autologous vs. alloplastic breast reconstructive surgery (Klasson, 2016). The perioperative period can thus be a teachable moment at least to counteract these smoking-related surgery risks, and what we know by now is that:

- Even light smoking associates a higher risk of wound dehiscence and infection after all types of surgery and of skin flap necrosis and epidermolysis after simple

mastectomy and modified radical mastectomy (Sørensen L. T., 2002).
- To decrease postoperative complication risks, smoking cessation should start at least one month before surgery (Wong J. e., 2012).
- There is no proof that quitting smoking shortly before surgery increases postoperative complications (Myers, 2011).
- Counseling and pharmacotherapy can increase the chance of abstinence maintenance by up to 60% within 3 to 6 months following surgery (Zaki, 2008).
- In RCTs with intensive, multicomponent interventions, 6 to 12-month abstinence rates topped 36.4% in RCTs with intensive, multicomponent interventions (Gavilan, 2023).

So, even with intensive, multicomponent interventions, at most, 4 in 10 people manage to remain tobacco abstinent at 12 months after surgery. And besides the overall unhealthy impact, why I care about smoking cessation as a clinical nutritionist doing supportive work in oncology is that in most clinical scenarios, both the healthcare providers and the patients initially overlook that smoking cessation frequently comes with weight gain. And then it blows up in all of our faces. And then most healthcare providers either do nothing about it or blame the patient for gaining weight. Patient or not, one gets fatter and fatter with any smoking cessation failed attempt; thus, the fear of weight gain remains a barrier to cessation, or it may lead to smoking relapse in those requiring but not having access to professional nutrition.

The curious thing about preventive smoking cessation weight gain interventions is that although they work, many concluded a long time ago that they aren't really worth the effort as they are only effective while they are followed.

Kind of like, if there is no "and then they lived happily ever after," why bother?! But is there anything on Earth with a "and then, they lived happily ever after" ending? And while this is an old view (Spring, 2009) confirmed by new eyes (García-Fernández, 2023), what would we expect to see when the recommendations are no longer followed? If yesterday you ate well and tonight you're binging on donuts, dead-tired, and fainted on your sofa, do you expect that what you did yesterday prevents you from gaining fat from what you do today?! Any nutritional intervention is effective only while it's followed.

The **MATCH** acronym summarizes why people gain weight when they try to stop smoking:

- **Metabolism** - while it is true that nicotine intake increases lipolysis, it also lowers muscular glucose uptake gradually, leading to insulin resistance (Bajaj, 2012). Insulin resistance is what remains when smoking cessation starts, which is one of the main causes of weight gain. Both metabolic syndrome risk (Kim H. J., 2024) and type II diabetes risk increase initially post-cessation in those gaining ≥2.0 kg (Wu L. e., 2022).
- **Appetite** - nicotine intake lowers food intake by direct impact on all hypothalamic areas involved in appetite control (Hu T. Z., 2018). This means that:
  - when you're hungry and you smoke, you may perceive being less hungry,
  - when you no longer smoke, you will become aware of your appetite on top of the amplified insulin resistance, thus have an increased tendency to eat more and gain fat unless you manage to control yourself and increase your muscle insulin sensitivity back by minding your food intake and by practicing physical exercises (Jain P. e., 2020).
- **Taste** - tobacco intake by smoking (Milani, 2023) or chewing (Kale, 2019) has a detrimental effect on taste

buds, and smoking cessation leads to a rapid recovery of taste sensitivity (Chéruel, 2017). Thus, on top of the amplified insulin resistance and increased appetite, initially, after you stop using tobacco, food will start to taste better.

- **Cravings** - psychosocial distress increases the desire to smoke, and the pleasure from smoking the first cigarette (Childs, 2010), and smokers high in social anxiety have a higher risk for ongoing smoking (Watson, 2018). If self-soothing by smoking is a go-to behavior under stress, this doesn't just go away on its own, being usually replaced with other coping behaviors. Eating is one of the easiest behaviors to cool things down under stress. Some people replace distress-smoking with distress-eating, then quit quitting smoking because of the weight gain. That is not to even mention that distress-smoking and binge eating frequently co-occur, and women with an eating disorder have a significantly higher motivation to smoke as a means of weight control and to cope with anxiety (Brachthäuser, 2024). However, the relationship between low distress tolerance and smoking is not set in stone, as it can be changed if it's intentionally worked on (Veilleux, 2019). And sports can help (Zheng, 2024). And psychotherapy can help (Lancaster, 2017). Nonetheless, it's important to keep in mind that besides all other detrimental impacts, smoking may also be associated with chronic dysbiosis (Cicchinelli, 2023), which lowers the inner ability to have patience while enhancing premature responding and impulsivity by the subsequent lowered serotonin (Worbe, 2014). Therefore, smoking cessation in people with a diagnosis and treatments with intestinal side effects may feel like they're fighting an uphill battle, potentially lost from the start at the intestinal level if antidepressive medications are not on the table (Shoaib, 2018).

- **Hand-to-mouth** - this is the last part of the smoking addiction to break, and many are not aware how a repetitive movement like the hand-to-mouth is part of the conditional reflex built into the ritual of smoking until they lose access to it. Some try to replace it by taking e-cigarettes (Lindson, 2024) or nicotine-free inhalators to the mouth (Shete, 2023), and some by food grazing (Bonder, "Associations between food addiction and substance-use disorders: a critical overview of their overlapping patterns of consumption.", 2022), replacement behaviors that keep the addiction on the table by enabling the hand-to-mouth self-calming ritual. The need to take something to the mouth when stressed is sometimes seeded by the childhood pacifier and thereafter groomed throughout the years of distress-smoking and compulsive grazing in a positive feedback loop that may never end (Bonder, 2022).

From the day one decides to quit smoking, the nutritional MATCH is on the table, and fat gain can happen regardless of the evolution of the total body weight. Thus the first thing to do about it is to understand, expect, and prepare for it. And while all these may feel discouraging, not quitting continues the many detrimental effects of smoking. Moreover, the hardship can be temporary, with successful smoking cessation being associated with improved distress tolerance and better mood, health, and quality of life when compared with those of people who continue to smoke (Taylor G. e., 2014).

The smoking cessation transition from current smoker to long-term non-smoker is like crossing the street: you can do it on your own whenever you feel like you're ready, attentive, and skillful enough to self-police, or you can look for a pedestrian crossing and wait for the green traffic light if you want to decrease the risk of crossing the street in a riskier way. And, of course, crossing a street and crossing a roundabout may be two completely different situations.

Without professional nutrition, physical exercise, psychological support, and sometimes also medication, many smokers become experts in smoking cessation techniques while repeatedly restarting to smoke, as this behavior is ingrained into the smoker's identity. If now you smoke, the longer you smoke, the more it becomes part of who you are as a person.

You are a smoker when you're stressed, when you're out with your friends, and when you take breaks during workdays. And you remain a smoker when you're sick, as a diagnosis doesn't include a personality transplant.

To quit for real, you must take ownership of your day-to-day behavioral choices in order to get out of the drama triangle and work through your personal issues enough to act resilient. And what you must face when deciding to quit is the loss of the emotional comfort you get from familiarity.

Intermittent compliance is founded on the need for the cortisol/dopamine binge when perceived inner power is low. Inconsistency is addictive as it builds up both the stress and the need to binge. Most people don't wake up in the morning asking how they can harm themselves better today. People smoke, drink, overeat, buy things they don't need when they're broke, and lose themselves in video games or pornography because they get something out of it at the moment.

Thus, if you smoke, instead of debating the carcinogenity of tobacco intake or the lack of impact on the oncology outcomes, maybe you could take a deep look at your life to acknowledge: What are the subjective benefits you actually get from smoking?

Until you'll acknowledge and get these from somewhere else, you'll remain attached to smoking.

The patient changes when she decides it's important enough for her to resist using it, that she's able to do it, and that there is no one to blame, save, or shame for not doing her part. Taking ownership is essential in all treatments self-administered by the patient, and smoking cessation is a treatment self-administered by the patient. A person in the pre-contemplation stage might even feel insulted by the unsolicited advice despite it coming from a professional. Thus, knowing where someone is before recommending a behavioral change is a step forward in becoming aware of the patient-related part of personalized medicine.

This is backed up by evidence, as RCTs comparing stage-matched vs. stage-mismatched smoking cessation interventions show that the matched interventions had twice the efficacy (Dijkstra, 2006). The link between patients' readiness to quit smoking and therapy outcomes was on the kitchen table all along while humanity trained astronauts to search for it in the sky. Just telling someone to do something will never work. Outcomes of any self-applied therapeutical intervention in free-living settings are a function of the pretreatment stage of change of the persons applying it; the farther along the stages, the better the outcomes (Krebs P. e., "Stages of change and psychotherapy outcomes: A review and meta-analysis.", 2018).

Even smoking clinicians from the multidisciplinary team treating smoking oncology patients find it hard to quit smoking, some bringing many reasons to support the supposed harmlessness of this self-soothing behavior, which basically helped them cope with stress. And it's not like change is hard for us because we're so busy and tired, while the patients will just do it. Changing an identity-ingrained behavior is hard for all of us. Thus, if we add the diagnosis and treatment-induced stress to the fact that smoking cessation in itself is stressful, patients with breast cancer who smoked before diagnosis must be elite ninjas at self-discipline to successfully stop smoking after diagnosis. And it looks like 6 out of 10 are not.

That is why—besides the physicians and the nurses—at least a clinical psychologist is an essential part of the multidisciplinary team when parts of the treatments are to be self-applied.

Chapter 8
Polypragmasia

Many people try to decrease cancer risk by taking all sorts of supplements promoted as "anticarcinogenic" in the hope that an increased immunity will defend them. Breast cancer patients are the champions of taking dietary supplements, with up to 84% of them taking such products without discussing them with any healthcare provider (Roumeliotis, 2017). However, immunity is a much more complex system than it seems when talking about it while having a Corona. And the main thing to keep in mind when leaning into natural polypragmasia is that dietary supplements are not medicines.[6] And no, this does not mean they don't have side effects because they're natural. Cocaine is natural, too.

What this means is that dietary supplements' side effects are less acknowledged because, by law, they are not evaluated for safety or efficacy, being produced and marketed according to regulations completely different from the ones used for medicines.

While nutrition might seem to fit into the pharmacological complementary therapies, professional nutrition is not about dietary supplements but about food. Real food. Normal food.

---
[6] https://www.efsa.europa.eu/en/topics/topic/food-supplements

Yummy food. Even in the case of blood test-proven deficiency, professional nutrition remains first and foremost about correcting the food intake and only second about carefully and temporarily recommending the lowest amount possible of the best proven dietary supplements financially and logistically available to each individual patient. We do not ignore the socioeconomic reality. We also work hand in hand with the treating physicians.

Physicians treat the patients.

Alongside clinical psychologists and physical therapists, dietitians do professional supportive care.

Unlike complementary medicine practitioners—coming from all walks of life with regard to any healthcare formal training—oncology dietitians are not natural healers who sprouted on the face of the planet to cure cancer in a natural way. Nevertheless, today, we're witnessing a full-blown inundation of self-named nutritionists, although, in most countries, this is a profession with formal university training.

To legally practice professional nutrition, one must graduate from the Nutrition and Dietetics Faculty and own a bachelor's and a master's degree in nutrition, not a certificate of "complementary medicine practitioner" or a "certificate of attendance" from a conference. The self-named "nutritionist" epidemic is flourishing worldwide because many people are confused about the fact that some physicians decided to mingle with the people practicing alternative "medicine" and by the many available unprofessional nutrition diplomas.

Practicing nutrition by having an unprofessional diploma includes the ESPEN lectures and classes, which are not meant to replace a bachelor's degree or to change one's profession into a thereafter self-proclaimed "nutritionist."

And although this gradually became more and more popular among physicians who are considering upgrading their practice with some nutrition too, all the way down to the LLL website, one can read that their Diploma in Clinical Nutrition and Metabolism is just a Continuing Medical Education endorsement "not an equivalent of a formal degree recognized by the Ministry of Education of any country."[7]

Professional boundaries are simply ignored by the physicians self-proclaiming themselves "nutritionists" simply because no one actually asked them about their nutrition-specific formal training. These people don't practice medicine and they don't practice nutrition, using people's trust in medicine to practice a profession they do not have.

And this behavior is not nutrition-specific. As Prof. Sam Vaknin says, "Information does not amount to knowledge. Curiosity and education are not one and the same. Anecdotes do not a science make. Experience is not a synonym for expertise."[8] Therapy-speak is abuse and manipulation exactly as the pseudo-nutrition practiced by people with no professional nutrition training.

This includes the physicians with no professional nutrition training projecting whatever subjective eating ideas they might have onto the more and more confused patients.

From self-proclaimed "psychotherapists" with zero psychology training, to "sport specialists" with no training in exercise physiology, to expert "photographs" by the virtue of owning an iPhone, nowadays everyone can seem an expert in anything. Long live the king of virtual perception throned on the Dunning-Kruger effect!

---

[7] https://lllnutrition.com/mod/page/view.php?id=3318
[8] https://www.youtube.com/watch?v=Gd3ahuCu-HY

But regardless of the confidence and enthusiasm of people who don't know how much they don't know, as David Dunning said long time ago, "Outside our field of expertise, we are all confident idiots." And what is kept aside in the attempt to somehow increase access to the supportive care professional areas of nutrition, physical therapy and psychology, is that practicing these unprofessionally can have side effects that can worsen patients' physical, mental and financial health.

Oncology nutrition requires one of the highest levels of both nutrition and oncology training as first we should do no harm. And to do no harm, we must have the level of knowledge necessary to understand the consequences of our recommendations. But in the today's complementary, alternative, pseudo-nutrition no man's land, many of the people recommending extreme diets or bucket loads of supplements to cancer patients do not understand how serious the consequences can be, both for the patient and for the other physicians working with the patient who might experience more side effects to a properly prescribed or applied treatment.

And not all physicians play "nutritionist."

And not all patients allow themselves to be played by "nutritionists." Those who do believe in shortcuts.

Just that there are no shortcuts in oncology.

RCT evidence proving dietary supplements implied lack of side effects is mostly missing, although these are typically prone to batch-to-batch variability in composition and concentration, contamination, and adulteration with undeclared substances.

Their popularity is based on the dietary supplements law, which is quite loose, on the fact that to bring such a product on the market one just has to fill up a paper, and on the marketing-built beliefs and hope (Hudson, 2018).

And, by law, regardless of who made the recommendation, the sole responsibility for the consequences of taking a dietary supplement or a herbal remedy is of the adult's freely choosing to take it—be them a healthy person or an oncology patient under active treatment—thus, to make an informed decision it is important to take into consideration two aspects:

Most dietary supplements are not tested for safety in oncology settings.

The main side effects of dietary supplements are their interactions with the medication, hepatic and renal injury, disordered coagulation, and autoimmunity.

Potential interactions between Cytochrome P450 enzyme activity and various dietary supplements' active substances and plant remedies phytochemicals can be checked on the Thériaque®,[9] German Pharmacopoeia,[10] Drugs.com®,[11] and Memorial Sloan Kettering Cancer Center (MSKCC)[12] databases.

This is important not only because these interactions may influence oncology medication pharmacokinetics but also because many herbal remedies sold on the seemingly free alternative "medicine" market have been linked to significant liver injury (Stickel, 2015).

Hepatic toxicity is one of the main side effects of dietary supplements (Navarro, 2014), with the individual herbs with the greatest reported liver toxicity being germander, black cohosh, kava, and green tea extract (Brown A. C., 2017).

---

[9] https://www.theriaque.org/
[10] https://arzneipflanzenlexikon.info/en/german-pharmacopoeia.php
[11] https://www.drugs.com/drug_interactions.html
[12] https://www.mskcc.org/cancer-care/diagnosis-treatment/symptom-management/integrative-medicine/herbs/search

Immune-mediated nephrotoxicity, acute renal injury, and hepatorenal syndrome are other potential side effects of dietary supplements (Brown A. C., 2017). Renal toxicity risk is higher for herbal remedies as soil contamination can lead to heavy metals bioaccumulation (Charen, 2020).

The main heavy metals of health concern are arsenic, cadmium, lead, and mercury, which can contaminate not only plant-based dietary supplements but also medicinal plant teas (de Oliveira L. M., 2018). In healthy people, drinking a couple of tea infusions per day does not exceed the critical levels established for the general population, as 65-80% of the toxic substances remain in the leaves after brewing. However, in oncology settings, moderation is prudent, and patients with pre-existing kidney disease or who developed renal side effects during systemic treatments need to be carefully evaluated by an oncology dietitian or by another healthcare provider formally trained in food toxicology (Grządka, 2024).

Disordered coagulation is another dietary supplement and plant remedy side effect important to remember, especially during breast cancer surgery and during medical oncology treatments with a higher risk of thromboembolic events.

Most of the available information on herbal remedies containing aloe, echinacea, ginseng, ginger, chamomile, and alfalfa is based on in vitro experiments, animal studies, and clinical case reports. And obviously, there is no need to worry about drinking chamomile tea in the morning. However, since these products are often self-administered, some patients can overdose to increase self-perceived natural protection and thereafter feel ill or experience bleeding and interpret it as a cancer treatment side effect (Gouws, 2020).

Patients may withhold important information from their clinicians and are most likely to do so when they disagree with, distrust them, or misunderstand their instructions (Levy A. G.,

2018). And since the effects of dietary supplements and herbal remedies on platelet function and anticoagulant medication are hard to predict, it is important to ask about and advise their discontinuation at least before surgery (Wang C. Z., 2015). Moderation is also wise in patients treated with CDK 4/6 inhibitors alongside antiestrogenic medications due to the higher thromboembolic risk (Bolzacchini, 2021). There are many cardio-oncology considerations that need to be closely monitored multidisciplinary in higher-risk patients (Beavers, 2022).

There is conflicting data on vitamin K intake from food sources' impact on coagulation, as some studies found a negative correlation with INR, while others suggest that a small amount of vitamin K is required to maintain adequate anticoagulation. But all this discussion is about food, as supplements can contain a hundred times higher amounts of active substances.

Vitamin K's influence on anticoagulant efficacy depends on each patient's vitamin K status, the intake amount, and the intake source—the impact being much higher for supplements than for foods. The intake of foods higher in vitamin K, like leafy green and cruciferous vegetables, is advisable to be low to moderate during such treatments, this being a general recommendation that must be individualized on a case-by-case basis (Violi, 2016).

Additionally, taking vitamin E alongside vitamin K supplements or alongside antithrombotic medication may have an increased bleeding effect by amplifying abnormal blood clotting (Shea, 2019). Many patients and some healthcare providers don't know about these interactions and take or recommend vitamin K supplements because they're known to contribute to bone health.

But, while it is true that vitamin K intake from foods is important for bone health, systematic review data shows no efficacy of vitamin K supplements for the prevention or treatment of osteoporosis (Mott, 2019).

Another important thing to keep in mind when considering taking dietary supplements to increase immunity is that many actually do increase immunity. And it might seem quite odd that taking dietary supplements specifically to increase immunity has increased immunity as a side effect. But the odd part is only for those thinking they can somehow buy immunity.

Many people have no clue about exactly what immunity is. The subliminal message passed on from one to another is that they must take vitamins, antioxidants, or something to better defend themselves against infections during treatment and/or against cancer coming back. Immunity is not a magical door toward better health but an entirely defensive system. And like any defense system, it's a huge system.

There are two things to know when it comes to messing with the immune system:

- The only part of the immune system that can be increased without disease, vaccines, or immunotherapy is nonspecific immunity. This is called nonspecific because it is nonspecific, making no difference between self and non-self. Thus, increased nonspecific immunity does not mean better defense and more health; it means military dictatorship with a higher risk of autoimmunity (Lucius, 2019).
- Before even talking about increasing immunity, maybe it would help to stop decreasing it. The anatomical, biochemical, and humoral barriers are the customs officers that the enemy must overcome to trespass into the human body. And even if it doesn't sound as fancy

as taking some exotic pills, the skin, the nose hair, the eyelashes, and the mucus on these digestive and respiratory membranes are the first defense against most infectious diseases. Then we have tears, saliva, blinking, coughing, sneezing, vomiting, low gastric pH, and intestinal peristalsis—all responsible for defending the body when under attack. If life is a ping-pong between fast food, soda drinks, low-quality sweets, laxatives, and detoxes sprinkled with holy vitamin C, the customs officers will not raise a finger to do their job when most needed. When you take no care of your customs officers, they will take no care of you. To empower customs officers, you need to do regular physical exercise, rest throughout the day, and make the required lifestyle changes to increase sleep quality, drink enough water, and have a healthy diet on a day-to-day basis.

A higher concentration of active substances is the foundation of the "more is better" marketing. However, a higher impact without toxicity data does not mean a better impact, but an uncontrolled, stronger one. And this uncontrolled, stronger impact can also be detrimental.

There is no clinical efficacy data for most dietary supplements.

Randomized controlled trials performed on supplements with vitamin B (Zhang S.-L. e., 2016), vitamin C (Lee B. S.-W.-K., 2015), vitamin D (Gallagher J. C., 2023), or vitamin E (de Oliveira V. A., 2024) are negative for cancer prevention. And, data on graviola (Ioannis, 2015), turmeric (Yang Z.-J. e., 2022), and indole-3 carbinol (Williams, 2021) are mainly preclinical, while the evidence for recommending medicinal mushrooms in oncology settings remains inconclusive (Narayanan, 2023).

There are many diseases called "cancer," and different cancers have multiple different causes that remain completely untouched by such panacea. There is no international consensus about what exactly "dietary supplements" are; these are legally defined in most countries by what they contain (Dwyer, 2018), not by what they do (Thakkar, 2020).

Despite biological plausibility being hypothesized based on preclinical and epidemiological data, it is almost impossible to assess the role of singular micronutrients and phytochemicals as these may also be consumed from legumes, grains, kernels, fruits, and vegetables, and it is difficult to discern how each separately influences the human body. Singling out this or that substance ignores that:

- the effect a substance has on cell lines or lab animals might not be the same after a human consumes that substance,
- the effect might be completely different from patient to patient based on individual factors that might not be taken into consideration when a supplement is generally prescribed (Rudzińska, 2023).

The panacea symbol is built on compelling abstract words that ignore the low-quality studies, their heterogeneity, and high bias. Furthermore, the negative results are sometimes replaced with subsequent reinterpretations of minute cancer survival differences, which are barely there even in underpowered studies.

For instance, many RCTs assessing the effect of vitamin D supplementation on cancer risk have been recently published despite the negative previous evidence stating that hypovitaminosis D is another one of the many consequences of an unhealthy lifestyle. Not the cause.

Both hypovitaminosis D and these illnesses are consequences. And the cause does not disappear by wiping away one of its consequences. Even vitamin D deficiency doesn't disappear when you take vitamin D supplements if you don't first have vitamin D deficiency.

The supplements' built-up health image contributes to the fact that in 2019, the sale of vitamin D supplements registered a profit of $ 1.1 billion, and the dietary supplement industry expects this profit to reach $ 1.9 billion in 2029.[13] And while this would make sense with safety and efficacy data, vitamin D supplement recommendations are not evidence-based but eminence-based, using mathematics, literature, and marketing.

For instance, the VITAL trial—applauded by some, tossed out by others, and reinterpreted thereafter in the attempt to get something out of its negative results—showed zero impact for 2000UI vitamin D or for 1g omega-3 fatty acids on preventing cancer of any type (Manson, 2019).

...but this was in people over 50.

Thus, other researchers from Finland tried their luck as well in another attempt to prevent complex pathologies like cancer and cardiovascular disease with the same panaceas, but this time in people over 65. The results were just as negative; after five years of 1600 IU/day, or 3200 IU/day vitamin D3, there was no cardiovascular protection and no impact on cancer incidence or mortality compared to placebo (Virtanen, 2022).

The D-Health RCT showed that supplementing unscreened adults with vitamin D did not reduce all-cause mortality, being associated with an increased risk of cancer-specific mortality (Neale, 2022).

Furthermore, without objectively proven deficiency, vitamin D supplementation doesn't improve musculoskeletal

---

[13] https://www.marketsandmarkets.com/PressReleases/vitamin-d.asp

health (Bolland, 2018), and it does not prevent osteoporosis (Reis, 2023). Nevertheless, in many breast cancer clinical settings, the deficiency is assumed instead of checked out on the patient's current blood tests.

It is so easy to take or to recommend supplements to others.

But for the past 100 years, RCTs showed no efficacy of vitamin D in preventing cardiovascular diseases, type 2 diabetes, asthma, respiratory infections, or cancer (Autier, 2017). And the same is true for all omega-3 fatty acids supplements' supposed benefits, with RCT data showing either little or no effect whatsoever for primary and secondary prevention of cardiovascular disease (Abdelhamid, 2018), anxiety or depression (Deane, 2021), Alzheimer's disease (Araya-Quintanilla, 2020), type 2 diabetes (Brown T. J., 2019), or inflammatory bowel disease (Ajabnoor, 2021).

Preclinical and epidemiological data build a world of assumptions based on peoples' unverified replies to questionnaires asking them what they ate three months or three years ago, although, if asked when they least expect it, most would not even remember what they ate three weeks ago.

Despite negative RCTs, based on preclinical and epidemiological data, vitamin D and omega-3 fatty acids have gradually become a health symbol, with many recommending them on autopilot with literally no scientific proof of efficacy.

Taking supplements is currently perceived as a health-promoting behavior that can replace the effort that's necessary to eat right, rest, learn to communicate effectively to keep calm, spend more time outside, and practice regular physical activity.

Things got to such a level of manipulative marketing that even on these products, it is written that taking them doesn't replace healthy eating or living. Still …you can take this supplement to keep calm, you can take that supplement to force yourself to sleep when emotionally under the weather, you can take the other supplement when you avoid whole categories of foods, and you can take the other supplements to increase metabolism when you don't feel like stopping being sedentary.

Opposite to hopeful preclinical and epidemiological correlations, RCT evidence continues to show that taking supplements doesn't offer any special benefits or protection besides correcting deficiencies if these deficiencies existed in the first place. And while many refuse to acknowledge the side effects of dietary supplements, they are there. One can mock science by inviting evidence-based nutrition fans to participate in a double-blind, randomized, placebo-controlled crossover trial to determine whether parachutes are effective in preventing major trauma related to gravity when jumping from an airplane.

The truth remains, though, that—even after a cancer diagnosis—many people would do close to anything except the actual work required to take care of the part of themselves they kept on overlooking. To eat right, do the sports, respect the sleep hygiene, improve assertiveness and conflict resolution skills, spend time outside in nature, and actually talk to people outside social media—nowadays, all seem like such a drudgery that you can easily replace unprofessionally.

Unfortunately, there is no magic pill.

Chapter 9
Veganism

A cancer diagnosis comes along with the juicer and *The China Study* book, frightened patients and many of the concerned caregivers reeling into popular natural ways to fight against the oncology treatments' horrors they've heard about, many being as or more afraid of the treatment as they are of the diagnosis. Like drowning people that fight the ones trying to get them out of the water, instead of helping us help them, some start fighting us. And whatever anyone working within the field of oncology might say, most of us haven't gone through chemotherapy, potentially identity-inflicting surgery, or radiotherapy in our lives, and each and every person tolerates these differently. While the fear is valid, defensiveness may ruin the chance to fix things, as the main shields promoted in oncology are:

- To load up on antioxidants = have an as high as possible intake of micronutrients.
- To avoid "animal protein" = have as little as possible intake of the main macronutrients needed in oncology: proteins.

Sometimes, even highly trained healthcare providers forget that our survival depends on macronutrients. A plant-based diet may have the potential for cardiometabolic disease prevention, but this is oncology. And in oncology settings, we work with people who already have a cancer diagnosis and preventing something vs. treating something are entirely different clinical scenarios.

The main thing to keep in mind in professional oncology nutrition is that to ensure proper metabolism throughout the many treatments, the muscle protein synthesis/muscle protein breakdown rate must be kept as even as possible (Gorissen, 2015), or the patient will go into muscle catabolism.

- **Muscle protein synthesis** is coamplified by proper protein intake (Prado, 2020) and regular physical activity (Li X. e., 2023).
- **Muscle protein breakdown** is amplified by chemotherapy (Godinho-Mota, 2021).

In general, vegans of any age need to eat more protein than recommended for omnivores because of the reduced plant protein digestibility (Agnoli, 2017). Despite common assumptions, proteins of animal origin are easier to digest and more absorbable, contributing to a more efficient prevention of muscle and bone loss (Beasley, 2013). Adequate nutrition alone cannot counteract the sedentariness-increased risk of muscle and bone loss, the regular practice of physical exercise being essential at any age, the main risk factors for frailty including age, malnutrition, and physical inactivity (Artaza-Artabe, 2016).

The current evidence from cohort studies shows that the complete exclusion of animal sources of protein from the diet is not associated with benefits for human health, even in healthy people (Godos, 2017).

This is not important only in premenopausal patients with cancer, who are frequently the ones who lose the most muscle if they don't have the knowledge or the discipline to take care of their muscle protein synthesis throughout treatments. This is also important in patients who were overweight or obese before the cancer diagnosis, as the anabolic sensitivity to consumed protein-dense food is reduced in overweight and obese young adults from the get-go (Beals, 2016). And this gets even more important in elderly patients, who are physiologically more resistant to the anabolic impact of protein and physical activity (Breen, 2011).

Geriatric nutrition is as much of a foreign concept for those who don't need geriatric nutrition as it is oncology nutrition for those who have nothing to do with oncology.

Based on the current evidence, the recommended protein intake in healthy older people is 1.0–1.2 g protein/kg of body weight/day, whereas the recommended protein intake for those who are malnourished or at risk of malnutrition due to acute or chronic illnesses is almost twice of that of a healthy adult, reaching 1.2–1.5 g protein/kg of body weight/day (Deutz, 2014).

The declining anabolic response to the ingested proteins, the higher protein intake necessary to prevent or to counteract sarcopenia, osteopenia, and the frailty physiologically associated with aging, and the muscle detrimental impact of systemic treatments are usually ignored in the day-to-day oncology practice as most healthcare providers have no recollection of none of these professional nutrition information (Bauer, 2013). And—if in a generally healthy elder, this can somehow get under the radar—things can get more serious if this elder is scheduled for surgery, and that is because wound healing requires a higher protein intake (Weimann, 2021).

Furthermore, the main foods consumed by many of the older cancer patients are not protein but carbohydrate food sources: bread, pasta, potatoes, sweets, and easier-to-chew fruits—both because these are easily available and because they match the common recommendation to avoid foods high in saturated fats for cardiovascular protection.

But in oncology settings, the general recommendation to "avoid foods high in saturated fats" literally translates to "eat less protein." The consequent insufficient protein intake and the compensatory excessive carbohydrate intake gradually lead to metabolic deregulations: hyperinsulinemia, insulin resistance, and dyslipidemia. While these metabolic deregulations can be addressed with specific medication, without a balanced diet, the medication alone just addresses the consequences while the underground root cause progresses.

We can obtain optimal muscle anabolism and proper wound healing from a varied diet that combines animal-based and plant-based proteins, just that animal-based foods must represent the majority of the protein intake (i.e., ≥65%) as translating cancer prevention recommendations to the clinical oncology nutrition required during cancer treatment is insufficient (Ford, 2022). It is true that some older patients sometimes avoid milk because of postprandial intestinal discomfort reasons and that about 70% of the elderly have lowered lactase secretion while they age. But the lowered lactase secretion does not necessarily mean clinical manifestations as only a third of the people with age-related lowered lactase secretion develop any symptoms.

Dairy products remain among the most easily digestible foods for the elderly, their exclusion amplifying the age-related and treatment-related loss of skeletal muscle mass and bone mineral density (Gallo, 2023).

Contrary to the viral hypothesis that "animal protein" feeds "cancer" built on *The China Study* book:

- there is more than one type of "animal protein," and
- there is more than one type of milk protein.

Even the results of the vegan biochemistry professor Colin Campbell, who authored this popular book, show the beneficial impact of casein intake. And the carcinogen had been aflatoxin all along (Svoboda DO, 1966). Not casein. The results of his preclinical study were that:

- mice fed with the 5% casein diet during aflatoxin administration developed severe hepatic lesions (hepatomegaly, cholangiofibrosis, bile duct proliferation) and
- mice fed with the 20% casein diet during aflatoxin administration developed rare hepatic lesions with no cholangiofibrosis or bile duct proliferation.

This was not a surprise for Campbell, as he had previously shown in another study—which he later ignored—that aflatoxin is much more carcinogenic if protein intake is low (Campbell, 1976). Even the actual epidemiological analysis quoted by Campbell as a basis for his book shows:

- a small correlation between eating protein food sources of animal origin and an overall 3% increased cancer-specific mortality and
- a bit higher correlation between eating protein food sources of vegetal origin and an overall 12% increase in cancer-specific mortality (Chen J, 1990).

Both of these results were not statistically significant.

According to this official database,[14] the inhabitants of the Tuoli region:

- had an average daily consumption of:
    o 865.5 g dairy products
    o 371.6 g wheat flour products
    o 121 g of meat

- consumed extremely rarely or not at all:
    o potatoes – 5-6 times a year
    o vegetables – twice a year
    o fruits – maximum once a year
    o legumes – never
    o nuts – never
    o eggs – never
    o fish – never
    o vegetable oil – never

These people from China lived with dairy, bread, and meat, most of them being shepherds. These shepherds with a daily medium intake of 865.5 g dairy/day had a mathematically calculated lower mortality risk than the vegans from the Huguan region, but both of these correlations did not meet statistical significance. Nevertheless, according to Campbell's reinterpretation: "Even relatively small intakes of animal protein were associated with adverse effects. And people who ate the most plant-based foods were the healthiest."

Leaving aside the fact that even Campbell's own preclinical studies showed that a low protein intake amplifies carcinogens' harmfulness, all the debate about the impact of a low or high casein intake moves the spotlight away from the fact that in this study, not one mouse developed cancer.

---

[14] https://archive.org/details/dietlifestylemor0000unse

The black-on-white text written by Campbell himself as the conclusion of his study is that the lesions developed by mice fed with the 20% casein diet "probably present a higher tendency toward malignant transformation," although just in the next paragraph, he states that "the majority of these lesions regressed back to normal tissue" and that "only some of these lesions probably can persist" (Appleton, 1983).

How on Earth is this study the scientific proof that "animal protein" is carcinogenic?

Reinterpreting the results of an epidemiologic analysis performed by others to fit your preconceived ideas seems somewhat benign because epidemiologic studies don't prove causality. But to back up personal beliefs contradicted by studies you personally authored seems bogus.

The Indian researchers Mathur and Nayak also found Campbell's reinterpretations bogus; thus, in 1989, they followed the same 5% and 20% casein diet protocol during aflatoxin exposure, not on mice, but on monkeys. Their results confirmed one more time what Campbell showed both in 1976 and in 1983. Casein confers hepatic protection and increases survival even in the presence of such a powerful carcinogenic substance as aflatoxin:

- Most monkeys fed with the 5% casein diet died before 70 weeks, not having the time to develop any tumors.
- The few monkeys fed with the 5% casein diet that survived more than 90 weeks developed preneoplastic hepatic lesions.
- Most monkeys fed with the 20% casein diet survived more than 90 weeks and didn't develop any preneoplastic lesions.

Unlike Campbell, whose studies showed the same protective effect of casein but chose to present the results as he thought fit, Mathur and Nayak concluded that protein-caloric malnutrition, along with the intake of foods contaminated with aflatoxin, contributes to the high incidence of hepatic cancer in the geographical areas where these two etiological factors coexist (Mathur, 1989).

Despite spending a life militating against "animal protein," the only associations Campbell could finally sustain had nothing to do with any animal protein but with cholesterol:

"Plasma cholesterol in the 90-170 mg/dl range is positively associated with most cancer mortality rates. Foods of animal origin contain cholesterol. Foods of plant origin do not contain cholesterol. Thus, even small increases in the consumption of animal-based foods are associated with increased disease risk."

Most people on the planet, including vegans, have total cholesterol higher than 90 mg/dl; thus, according to Campbell, we're pretty much doomed since birth simply by being human. Nevertheless, many of the people who feel doomed after receiving a cancer diagnosis also feel the need to make extreme dietary changes, following his lead in the desperate attempt to do all they possibly think it is needed to contribute to their healing. However, taking things to extremes does not improve health.

When people stop eating "animal protein," the alternative protein source used instead is frequently soy. And soy has been one of the most controversial protein food sources for a very long time, both when it comes to the efficacy and safety of its estrogenic impact and when it comes to its protein capacity to counteract the muscle protein catabolism associated with aging and with oncology treatments.

The efficacy and safety of soy estrogenic impact is primarily related to isoflavones' similar structure to that of 17β-estradiol. The main soy isoflavone with estrogenic impact is considered to be genistein, although there is also conflicting preclinical data about daidzein, equol, and formononetin (Zhao T.-T. e., 2019).

What we know about the estrogenic impact from retrospective data and preclinical studies is that:

- The decreased breast cancer risk is associated only with soy consumption during childhood, before adolescence—when genistein acts like an estrogen antagonist (Korde, 2009).
- The increased risk is associated with soy consumption by menopausal women—when genistein acts like an estrogen agonist (Ju, "Genistein stimulates growth of human breast cancer cells in a novel, postmenopausal animal model, with low plasma estradiol concentrations." , 2006).

Retrospective data and preclinical data hold no causal value, though.

The old and new human studies that analyzed the outcome of soy intake from diet and dietary supplements in healthy women reached contradictory results, but of small magnitude of impact in either direction:

- The intake of dietary supplements with soy isoflavones over nine months in 24 non-Asian premenopausal women generated an increased estradiol blood level and the appearance of mammary hyperplastic epithelial cells (Petrakis, 1996).
- The intake of dietary supplements with soy isoflavones over 14 days in 80 premenopausal women had a weak

estrogenic impact on the mammary gland (Hargreaves, 1999).
- A systematic review of 8 RCTs with a duration of at least eight months shows that soy intake does not influence breast density in menopausal women, being associated with a small increase in breast density in premenopausal women (Hooper, 2010).
- A systematic review of 18 RCTs investigating the impact of soy food or supplements in daily amounts widely ranging from 36.5–235 mg/day for a period of 1–36 months found neither a detrimental nor a protective impact on breast density, estrogens, including precursors, metabolites, or estrogen response such as length of menstrual cycle, and markers of proliferation and inflammation (Finkeldey, 2021).

Some scholars' answer to this data was that the protective impact might be more obvious in Asian women, unlike in women living in Europe or the US (Chen M. e., "Association between soy isoflavone intake and breast cancer risk for pre-and post-menopausal women: a meta-analysis of epidemiological studies.", 2014), while others answered that the soy dietary exposure in Europe is lower than 1 mg/day as compared to the far higher amounts used in the studies which make their conclusion irrelevant for a real-world clinical impact. Data on Asians shows that less than 10% of people consume as much as 25 g of soy protein or 100 mg of isoflavones per day (Messina M. C., 2006). An analysis performed on 300,000 women aged 30–79 from 10 regions across China shows a mean soy isoflavones intake of only 5.4 mg/day soy isoflavones (Wei Y. e., 2020).

Here, we stumble again on the old academic excitement vs. clinical requirement for accurate scientific data necessary to make professional recommendations.

Neither observational (Wei Y. e., 2020) nor RCT data found conclusive evidence for soy isoflavones in decreasing breast cancer risk, even in Asia (Tang, 2012). EFSA panel, analyzing the scientific literature, concluded that it was not possible to derive a single evidence-based guideline, neither for the efficacy of bone density maintenance nor for the reduction of vasomotor symptoms associated with menopause (EFSA, 2012). And nor for the safety of soy isoflavones (EFSA, 2015). Although the mathematically calculated correlative numbers between soy isoflavone and a wide range of health outcomes are found to be statistically significant, these are unlikely to be causal as in non-Asian, non-vegetarian populations, the dietary exposure is too low for isoflavones to exert any physiological effects (Messina M. V., 2024).

Are the promoted health benefits real, or is soy just another overstretched health symbol?

Besides the irrelevantly high soy isoflavone doses used in trials vs. the real-world intake, soy impact may also be blurred by two additional factors:

- Soy-based foods available in Europe and America are usually ultra-processed (soy sausages, soy hamburgers, soy schnitzels, etc.), while Asians usually eat unprocessed soy. Thus, in Europe and the US, substituting animal-based with plant-based alternatives may not improve the diet (Katidi, 2023).
- Women living in Asia seem to have an overall healthier lifestyle than those living in Europe and the US: less sedentariness, less obesity, giving birth at more physiological ages, and less hormonal replacement therapy use (Chen M. e., 2014). Sadly, the gradual adoption of the Westernized diet and lifestyle has started to have a detrimental impact even in Asia.

Additionally, another issue overlooked since like forever is the assumed sameness of these foods. For instance, an analysis of the actual content of 85 samples of 40 different brands of soy milk performed over a three-year period showed that:

- the total isoflavone content varied by up to 5-fold among different commercial soy milk and was not consistent between repeat purchases,
- the ratio of genistein to daidzein isoflavone was higher in isolated soy protein-based versus whole bean soy milks, the greatest variability in isoflavone content being observed among brands of whole bean soy milks, and
- concentrations differed markedly between the soy protein isolates, varying by 200-300% (Setchell, 2003).

Thus, what exactly is "soy milk"? And what do we actually see when scholars gloss over such high-measured differences to make estimated calculations convenient?

Based on the available scientific data, professionally, we cannot either encourage or discourage healthy women from eating whole soy-based food for any health outcome. And what remains to be elucidated is if the recommendation of a potentially protective single dietary factor from the whole culinary tradition and lifestyle of the Asian women living in Asia is efficient enough to have a health impact on women with quite different lifestyles.

The lack of high-quality scientific data is also present in studies evaluating soy intake impact in patients with breast cancer.

Preclinical data on mice with ER+ tumors indicates a potential oncological risk associated with dietary supplements with genistein:

- Genistein stimulates breast tumors' growth in a dose-dependent manner (Allred, 2001).
- Genistein can reverse the inhibitory effect of letrozole on tumor growth and adversely impact breast cancer therapy (Ju, 2008).
- Genistein can generate Tamoxifen resistance because it can bind to the same estrogen receptors as this medication (Du, 2012).
- Genistein stimulates aromatase, potentially associating resistance to aromatase inhibitors treatment (van Duursen, 2011).

For patients with breast cancer, we have:

- conflicting epidemiological, food frequency questionnaire data:
    o Two epidemiological studies which conclude that soy intake in breast cancer patients is associated with decreased mortality based on results that are statistically non-significant both in non-Asian (Caan, 2011) and in Asian populations (Nechuta S. J., 2012)
    o Consuming whole soy-based foods does not increase recurrence risk in patients with ER+ breast cancers, but it may increase the risk of cancer recurrence in patients with HER2+ breast cancers (Woo, 2012).
- some short-term RCTs with inconsistent results:
    o In a mixed group of 45 women with benign and malignant breast tumors, the intake of dietary supplements with soy isoflavones for two weeks stimulated breast lobular proliferation (McMichael-Phillips, 1998).
    o The intake of soy isoflavones supplements for two weeks in 17 patients with breast cancer did not stimulate or inhibit proliferative changes in the mammary gland (Sartippour, 2004).

- A study on 140 patients with ER+ and ER- breast cancers who received dietary supplements with soy isoflavones for three weeks (from diagnosis to surgery) shows that genistein may cause genetic modifications that stimulate cellular proliferation (Shike, 2014).

Everyone can conclude exactly what they choose to conclude from these studies.

For professional nutrition clinical practice, though, we don't have enough efficacy and safety data to recommend soy in breast cancer settings (Rabelo, 2024).

And leaving aside the highly debated estrogenic impact of soy, in oncology settings, we need to keep sarcopenia in mind in all patients with treatments with muscular side effects or during surgical treatments, as when the patient eats too little protein, the insufficient intake gets compensated by muscle loss.

When it comes to muscle protein synthesis efficiency, not all animal-based proteins are the same, milk proteins having the highest protective muscular impact even when compared to the ones in meat.

Both soy and milk provide complete proteins, but different in terms of amino acid profile, digestibility, and intestinal absorption kinetics. As compared to whey, soy contains a lower quantity of essential amino acids on a per-gram basis and notably fewer branched-chain amino acids (van Vliet, 2015). The other plant-based proteins have lower digestibility and lower leucine content and are deficient in essential amino acids such as lysine and methionine, which compromise the complete amino acid profile required for muscle protein synthesis.

This lower anabolic capacity can be compensated for in healthy people by combining various plant-based proteins to provide a more favorable amino acid intake (Nichele, 2022). But to say that this is enough for people with cancer is an extrapolation, as based on the available scientific evidence, there is no proof that an exclusive plant-based protein intake is enough to prevent either the primary (age-related), or the secondary (cancer- or oncology treatment-related) sarcopenia (Berrazaga, 2019).

This is especially important in the elderly, as in their cases, both of these types of sarcopenia can be amplified in patients with too low protein intake by the reduced response to protein ingestion (Breen, 2011). When consuming the same exact amount of calories and the same exact amount of proteins from an omnivore vs. a vegan meal, the vegan meal fares far worse when it comes to muscle protein synthesis (Pinckaers, 2023). And we have muscle biopsy data showing that a whole-food omnivorous meal containing lean beef results in a greater postprandial muscle protein synthesis when compared with an isocaloric and isonitrogenous whole-food vegan meal even in healthy, older adults. Why would we risk lower muscle protein synthesis in the sick ones?

Moreover, in a vegan diet, obtaining sufficient intake and actual bioavailability of some macro- and micronutrients is difficult or impossible, the most critical being the essential amino acids and the B12 vitamin. Regarding macronutrients, vegan diets are lower in protein intake compared with all other diet types. Regarding micronutrients, vegan diets have no B12 vitamin unless fortified foods or dietary supplements are used and are low in B2, B3, and D vitamins and in iodine, zinc, calcium, potassium, and selenium (Bakaloudi, 2021). Consequently, the nutritional needs of pregnant and lactating women, infants, children, and adolescents (Richter M. e., 2016), and people of all ages diagnosed with chronic diseases and cancer, are not properly covered through a vegan diet.

For people diagnosed with all sorts of cancers, even a well-thought, properly cooked, whole-food vegan diet can:

- **Amplify muscle loss**, both age-related (Domic, 2022) and oncology-related (Calvani, 2023).
- **Impair bone health** (Selinger, 2023). Studies consistently show that vegans have a higher risk of fracture (Ogilvie, 2022); thus, vegan diets should be contraindicated in people at risk for osteoporosis and in healthy people they should be thoroughly planned to avoid negative consequences on bone health due to their lower bioavailability of bone-important macro- and micronutrients and the higher content of antinutrients (Iguacel, 2019). If the patient wants to or is recommended to lose weight, things can get from bad to worse fast as caloric restriction in a vegan diet may worsen bone health even more, lowering bone mineral density and increasing osteoporosis and fracture risk (Veronese, 2019).
- **Amplify neuropathy, chemo brain, cognitive dysfunction, and depression** as many people diagnosed with cancer stop taking their B12 supplements because they're afraid of the popular theory stating that "B vitamins feed cancer" (Zhang S.-L. e., 2016). And if this happens in older patients, the B12 deficiency can further amplify sarcopenia (Bulut, 2017).

The World Health Organization recommends a daily intake of 25 g of dietary fibers, an amount easily reached by consuming 2-3 fruits, a vegetable salad, or a portion of raw seeds or cooked legumes. However, some epidemiologic analyses show we can obtain a 4% breast cancer risk decrease for every 10 g of dietary fibers consumed daily—a correlation with no causal value meant to promote the intake of vegetal foods, not to recommend an excessive dietary fiber intake (Chen S. e., 2016). And although no clear threshold defines an excessive intake, most people experience intestinal discomfort around an intake of 50-75 g of daily dietary fiber intake: abdominal cramps, bloating, flatulence, steatorrhea, diarrhea, or constipation (Ho K.-S. e., 2012).

Behavioral-induced constipation is often caused by dehydration, insufficient or excessive consumption of dietary fiber, sedentariness (in free-living people), or immobility (in hospitalized patients). And even in this case, the recommendation remains moving from too high or from too low toward moderation:

- **Hydration** – drinking one glass of water soon after waking up and then 4-8 glasses of water throughout the day (Sayuk, 2023).
- **Dietary fiber intake** – three simple habits by which we can provide a proper supply of dietary fiber to counteract mild constipation are: eating whole grain products or cereals on a daily basis, eating fruits (not juicing them), and avoiding peeling fruits and vegetables. However, for more severe constipation, scientific data, and clinical practice suggest a closer look at the soluble vs. insoluble fiber intake:
    o **Moderate intake of foods high in soluble fibers** – can increase stool frequency: plums, apples, pears, oranges, compote, jam, barley, oats, etc. (Yang J. e., 2012).
    o **Low-moderate intake of foods high in insoluble fibers** –here we have conflicting data, some showing that these can aggravate constipation: wheat bran, whole wheat bread and pasta, legumes, kernels, seeds, and potatoes (Suares, 2011).
    o **Caution is recommended when considering dietary supplements with fibers or prebiotics** – as the available data has a high risk of bias, and these can also aggravate constipation, abdominal cramps, and bloating (Christodoulides, 2016).

- **Physical exercise** – is required in the prevention and treatment of constipation, and none can work without the other. Nutrition alone is not effective in sedentary patients, and sports alone is inefficient when hydration and nutrition are inadequate (Li Y. W.-D., 2021).

For the general healthy and physically active population, the moderate intake of these foods on a daily basis can be one of the foundational behaviors that sustain human health (Arayici, 2023). Vegetables, legumes, and whole cereals are an important part of a healthy eating plan as they provide proteins, carbohydrates, fats, vitamins, and minerals, but their excessive intake is not more beneficial because the main thing that influences their metabolic impact is the dietary fibers.

And while it is understandable that in oncology people look for the highest natural protection possible, moving the focus too far on the plant-based side increases the dietary intake of fibers, phytates, oxalates, polyphenols, and other plant components that inhibit iron and calcium absorption. For instance, excessive intake of whole soybean products (Lynch, 1994) or even excessive intake of whole grains (Ahmed A. M., 2014) can lower iron bioavailability. This side effect happens either through frequent excessive dietary intake or fiber supplements without adequate water intake and/or physical activity.

For healthy people who are not children, adolescents, pregnant or lactating women, a well-thought, properly cooked, whole foods vegan diet may be somewhat protective against cardiovascular disease as compared to the popular fast-food culture. And while the "more is better" mindset seems inborn in consumerist societies, putting an equal between "plant-based" and veganism is like putting an equal between moderation and extremes.

People are encouraged to think that if it's from plants, it's all safe because it's natural, as if animals were made by aliens. Tobacco is natural, too, as opposed to the artificially sweetened soft drinks and the margarine consumed by many vegans trying to convince others of the benefits of the implied healthier lifestyle in a manner that looks a lot like promoting adherence to a religion.

Nowadays, being a vegan has become so popular that for some, it has become a matter of personal identity, a symbol of superiority built on extremism (Bali, 2023). However, the psychological need to take things to extremes is not a manifestation of health, whereas the complete elimination of meat or animal products is not necessary either for cancer (Godos, 2017) or for cardiovascular disease prevention (Termannsen, 2022).

The higher purity of plant-based vs. animal-based foods concept ignores that plants can contain antibiotics, fertilizers, insecticides, fungicides, and all sorts of other residual pharmaceutical pollutants used in agriculture, thus we need moderation (Nguyen, 2023). And even though these are so blamed, when they are properly used in agriculture they are used for good reasons, not only for the food industry but also for human health.

Those believing that organic plant foods are safer do so despite the fact that the control of aflatoxins from bacterial contamination is difficult in organic farming, aflatoxins remains a group 1 human carcinogen.

There is much scientific debate on the validity of the benefits of organic health claims since there is no evidence showing a clear difference in the nutritional quality, safety, or health outcomes between conventionally grown and organic-grown plant foods (Giampieri, 2022).

And, for instance, we have data showing that a diet focus on organic vegetal foods is not associated with decreased breast cancer risk (Bradbury, 2014), while a multicenter hospital-based study performed in eight cancer centers in India shows that lifelong exposure to a vegan diet has little, if any, effect on the risk of breast cancer (Gathani, 2017).

The truth remains that although there are many unhealthy ultra-processed foods out there, they can come be both animal- and plant-based. The assumption that the metabolic effect of a food is solely related to the animal origin ignores details like:

- Baked potatoes, chips, French fries, and store-bought frozen or homemade mashed potatoes, either from real potatoes or from dehydrated potato flakes, are collectively perceived as the same potato potahto (Jaiswal, 2020).
- French fries fried in soybean oil, rapeseed, or palm oil are all called "French fries" (Chen J. e., 2022).
- Balanced omnivore diets are associated with the lowest consumption of all types of ultra-processed foods, be they of vegetal or animal origin (Ohlau, 2022). Here, we go back to the professional nutrition appeal to moderation as the higher the avoidance of animal-based foods, the higher the ultra-processed food consumption seems to get (Gehring, 2021).

In *The Risks and Benefits of a Vegan Diet* study, nearly all vegans consumed supplements (Weikert, 2020). Thus, not only people considering veganism in oncology settings need to read the supplements' labels and the supplements law that clearly states that supplements should not replace a healthy diet. Without supplements/fortified foods, severe vitamin B12 deficiency may occur, alongside calcium, vitamin D, vitamin A, omega-3 fatty acids, iron, zinc, selenium, iodine, and protein insufficiency (Koeder, 2024).

But supplements are not enough to cover all the nutritional deficiencies associated with a vegan diet. For instance, while vitamin B12 status can be similarly good in vegans and non-vegans with supplementation, in one-third of vegans iodine excretion is lower than the <20 μg/L threshold value for severe iodine deficiency (Weikert, 2020).

And completely leaving aside the lower digestibility and the gastrointestinal discomfort, during many of the cancer treatment days, the last thing the patient has time or is in the mood for is to plan, buy, and cook a highly complex, properly combined, whole-food vegan diet. In clinical practice, we need to remember that despite the selective reporting and the flamboyant cause-and-effect statements of the abundant observational data, both a vegan or an omnivore diet can be healthy or unhealthy according to the quality of the usually eaten foods. Although popular, calling a diet "healthy" because it is plant-based is not scientifically accurate.

Chapter 10

Alkaline diet

Some believe they can prevent or cure cancer by following an alkaline diet or by drinking alkaline water. Far more think that the alkaline diet is veganism vs. an omnivore approach, promoting it as an attempt to somehow make people eat more fruits and veggies. And if we look at the statistics showing that in the US, only 1 out of 10 adults barely eats two fruits per day, the attempt is valid (Lee-Kwan, 2017). However, the alkaline diet is a form of veganism elevated to a higher level of extremism, being built on a mathematical model that ignores upfront both food biochemistry and human physiology.

Alkalosis is promoted as healthy for humans and acidosis as unhealthy. However, the concept ignores that foods contain fat, carbs, and fibers solely because these nutrients are not part of the used mathematical equations in this abstract mathematical model. Based on the mathematical equations, foods are labeled:

- **"alkaline"** when they contain potassium, magnesium, or calcium: fruits and vegetables,
- **"acidic"** when they contain protein, phosphorus, or sulfate: meat, fish, seafood, eggs, dairy, almonds, kernels,

seeds, cornflakes, white bread, whole wheat bread, oats, rye, and all other whole grain cereals (Frassetto, 2007).

In the attempt to promote a higher fruit and vegetable intake, have we replaced human physiology and food biochemistry with marketing and search engine optimization so everyone would have it easy? Can we just simplify things so much in the name of good intentions?

In the current ways nutrition is practiced worldwide, everyone seems free to reinterpret things as they please. However, if we follow the actual working definitions in the book, the alkaline diet is a version of vegan diet based solely on fruits and vegetables (Vincent-Johnson, 2023).

And if in the context of veganism we can at least talk about the lower efficacy of plant-based proteins to maintain an adequate muscle protein synthesis/ muscle protein breakdown rate as even as possible, avoiding "acidic" food directly leads to muscle loss by the almost inexistent protein intake. Thus even considering the alkaline diet in oncology settings is an upfront prescription for protein energy malnutrition. Nevertheless, since nothing is actually measured—the alkalinity literature being based on calculated estimations—this became overtime a very cheap way to publish something. And here we stumble again on popular trends built on availability bias.

The abundant alkaline literature is based on correlational studies with the following steps:

- People willing to respond are given questionnaires asking about what they ate yesterday, two weeks ago, or throughout the last year (Cui, 2023).
- Then, a nutrient ratio is estimated by correlating these responses to databases, while, for instance, even assessing the phosphorus content of foods based on the

- available food databases is merely an estimation (Hannah, 2018).
- Then, mathematically imprecise equations are used to estimate renal excretion (Parmenter B. H., 2017).
- Then, the calculated value of the urine alkalinity is correlated with past, current, or future health without any consideration for human physiology (Ring, 2017).

The studies correlating food pH with health outcomes don't measure food intake in any real way.

Food databases' accuracy is implied, while quality control remains largely uncovered worldwide.

It is not the food alkalinity that is correlated with health; the calculated urine alkalinity is the factor that is correlated with health. Many researchers plead to at least include actual urinary measurements into the PRAL (potential renal acid load) and NEAP (net endogenous acid production) estimations before drawing conclusions between the diet-dependent acid-base load and human health (Parmenter B. H., 2020). But making such measurements has an actual cost and those who refuse to pay it do it based on the fact that it has been considered for a long time that overadjusting the self-declared food intake data is enough for a reasonable proxy (Gannon, 2008), although overadjustment is a high source of bias (van Zwieten, 2024). Nonetheless, the actual net acid excretion measured as the sum of urine ammonium and titratable acidity in 24-hour urines from 980 participants in the Chronic Renal Insufficiency Cohort study—where this theoretical concept might have a clinical point—showed no association between the calculated expectations and the actual measurements (Scialla, 2017).

Not only that the fat, carbs, or fibers' impact on human health is left aside, and nutrients' bioavailability is bluntly ignored by this mathematical model, but it also completely ignores that in a human body the up or down pH modifications are counteracted by digestive, sanguine, osseous, pulmonary, and renal pH buffering systems. The notion that consuming food with a low pH outside the body leads to a decrease in the pH inside the human body is contradicted by our physiology.

Among the many ions, there are two that influence blood pH: H^+ and HCO_3^-:

- When blood H^+ increases, pH decreases = the blood becomes acidic.
- When blood HCO_3^- increases, pH increases = the blood becomes alkaline.

But this is only temporary until the next buffering system is crossed by the continuously flowing blood. And the blood continuously flows throughout all these pH buffering systems, again, and again, and again, as a living human body self-regulates pH again, and again, and again.

The pH modifications unrelated to the eaten food are compensated by the fact that carbonic anhydrase makes H^+ and HCO_3^- into H_2CO_3, which further separates into CO_2 and H_2O based on physiological needs. And yes, we breathe out CO_2 and urinate H_2O in the most natural way possible, without the help of any diet, alkaline water, or sophisticated alkalinization device. Simply from God All Mighty.

The digestive pH buffering system keeps pH between normal ranges when we eat mixed meals made, for instance, of meat and rice or of almonds and fruits—both generating digestive juice secretion:

- gastric juice high in H^+,
- pancreatic juice high in HCO_3.

Proteins from meat or almonds' digestion are initiated by gastric juice. To secrete gastric juice, H^+ is taken from the blood into the gastric cells, while HCO_3^- is taken from gastric cells into the blood. This ionic exchange determines a physiological alkalinization of the blood at the gastric level.

So, the digestion of food with an acidic pH measured outside the human body—like meat—causes the blood to become more alkaline at the gastric level. The blood that leaves the stomach area is more alkaline when we eat meat than when we eat fruits. Any fruits.

Carbohydrate digestion from cooked starch in rice or from raw starch in fruits needs pancreatic amylase from the pancreatic juice. To make pancreatic juice, HCO_3^- is taken from the blood into the pancreatic cells, while H^+ is taken from the pancreatic cells into the blood, which leads to the neutralization of the alkalinized blood that came from the stomach.

So, a food with an alkaline pH measured outside the human body—like fruits—causes the blood to acidify at the pancreatic level. The blood that leaves the pancreatic area is more acidic when we eat fruits without nuts. Any nuts.

The recommendation to eat fruit alone, as a snack between meals ignores how digestion runs physiologically in the human body, as the co-ingestion of other foods does not influence the digestibility of the fruit:

- The digestion of raw starch occurs in the small intestine, not in the mouth or the stomach. Pancreatic amylase is the only enzyme responsible for the digestion of the raw starch found within fruits—pancreatic juice containing all enzymes necessary to digest a mixed meal, including fruits: amylase, proteases, and lipases (Whitcomb, 2007).

- People perceiving that eating fruits with meals makes these ferment in the stomach don't know or ignore that without a gastric infection, the bacteria that could ferment the carbohydrates are missing from the stomach under physiological conditions. Thus, if the symptoms do occur, a Helicobacter Pylori test is indicated as literally almost half of the world population is infected, increasing the risk of gastric cancer (Chen Y.-C. e., 2024).
- In the absence of a gastric infection, fructose maldigestion generated by dysbiosis or intestinal dysmotility may cause abdominal discomfort—the cause being the damaged small intestine mucosa or irritable bowel syndrome, not the eating of the fruit as part of the meal which is only an effect. Thus, in patients with gastrointestinal symptoms, the cause needs to be addressed jointly by a gastroenterologist and a clinical nutrition specialist instead of covering things up by avoiding eating fruits as part of a meal (Jayasinghe, 2024).

When we consume mixed meals made of proteins and carbohydrate dietary sources, blood pH is physiologically neutralized right from the digestive buffering system. Thus, please do not eat meals or snacks made only of fruits; eat some protein sources along with the fruits, like some delicious pistachio or cashew nuts. And if you have symptoms when you eat fruits alongside other foods, go to the gastroenterologist.

Vegetables are healthy for us, but no proof exists that excessive intake increases protection. For instance, indole-3-carbinol—one of the more than 100 glucozinates found in cauliflower, broccoli, white or Brussels sprouts—is converted in the stomach to several compounds, including diindolylmethane and preclinical data show that this conversion can shift the metabolism of 17-βestradiol from 16-αhidroxiestrone toward 2-

hidroxiestrone. 16-αhidroxiestrone can be genotoxic (Fowke et al., 2000), but this preclinical hypothesis is used to market dietary supplements with indole-3-carbinol with no clinical proof of efficacy or safety (Amare, 2020).

We do not know the long-term effects of consuming dietary supplements with indole-3-carbinol. For breast cancer prevention, we recommend the moderate intake of cruciferous vegetables and against the more is better mantra used to sell supplements. And it is important to underline that consuming broccoli or other cruciferous vegetables is not correlated with overall survival or with recurrence risk after a breast cancer diagnosis (Nechuta S. e., 2013).

Another example is organosulfur compounds and selenium in garlic, a popular food among patients with cancer. But despite the high popularity built on the anticarcinogenic mechanisms suggested by preclinical studies (Tsubura, 2011), the studies that analyzed the impact of alliaceous vegetables' intake by humans show no clear evidence for a decreased breast cancer risk in healthy persons (Kim J. Y., 2009), researchers suggesting that the inconsistent evidence for garlic prevention of the stomach, breast, and prostate cancers may be explained by the manner of preparation or by different types of garlic (Farhat, 2021). Besides the many preclinical hypotheses, there is no human data proving the existence of an anticarcinogenic vegetable (Rudzińska, 2023).

Fruits are healthy for us, but there is also no proof that an excessive intake increases protection. For instance, the studies that analyzed the correlation between fruit intake and breast cancer risk show a relative risk of 0.93, interpretable by whomever in whatever way possible (Farvid M. S., 2021). People who like health symbols seem to look even for mere benefits to prove themselves right and then act surprised by the difference between the well-intended estimations and actual reality where ineffectiveness strikes.

The hope that things would be better if we somehow promoted it better is day-by-day becoming a toxic hope, while the planet is more and more confused by the many contradictory eminence-based opinions endorsed without actual evidence. With or without an impact on breast cancer, or any other cancer risk, fruits remain healthy foods that are high in carbohydrates, vitamins, minerals, dietary fibers, and phytochemicals, which have a beneficial impact on health.

Fruits seem important even for our mental health, interventional studies showing that the consumption of two servings of fresh fruits and vegetables per day contributes significantly to improving mood, personal satisfaction, happiness, and well-being (Conner, 2017). This study was performed in young adults, but it is a little piece of RCT data in a sea of epidemiological observations.

Like any other food, though, fruits must also be consumed in moderation. When the "more is better" is on the table, it is important to know that fructose has a different metabolism than glucose starting from the intestinal level, where it can be absorbed both through the glucose transporter (GLUT2) and through its own transporter (GLUT5). GLUT5 functions without ATP consumption; thus, fructose is completely absorbed no matter how much we consume, as humans don't have any mechanism to stop intestinal absorption in case of excessive fructose consumption (Ferraris, 2018). With a moderate intake of 2-3 fruits/day consumed at the end of a meal, as dessert, or as a mid-afternoon snack alongside some yogurt or nuts, the small quantity of fructose is used as the main energy source by small intestinal cells. The liver and kidney cells are the only other cells with the necessary enzymes to obtain energy from fructose (fructokinase and aldolase B).

Another issue, besides the required enzymes possessed by very few types of cells, is that fructose can be used for energy production only when there is no glucose in that cell.

Fruits contain a mix of fructose and glucose, which is why in the case of excessive intake of fruits—especially fruit juice which contains fewer dietary fibers, thus more rapidly absorbable fructose (Gonzalez, 2024)—the liver transforms the excess remaining from enterocytes by de novo lipogenesis into very low-density lipoproteins (VLDL) and triglycerides, with a side production of uric acid (Tappy, 2017). Consequently, excessive fruit intake—either as frequent or excessive fruit juice consumption, as meals made only of fruits, or nibbling fruits between meals throughout the day—can have a detrimental effect because of the way fructose is metabolized, potentially leading to dyslipidemia with hypertriglyceridemia, hyperuricemia, insulin resistance, and deregulated appetite.

Furthermore, excessive fruit consumption may not be detrimental only from a metabolic viewpoint but also from a pharmacological viewpoint. It is known that significantly more herbal-drug interactions occur in people trying to compensate for an exclusively vegan diet with herbal remedies and dietary supplements (Jermini, 2019). Grapefruit juice is a commonly known example of herbal-drug interactions, increasing plasma concentration and bioavailability of more than 50% of prescription drugs metabolized by CYP3A4. Other fruit juices can also induce herbal-drug interactions, leading to:

- **decreased drug bioavailability:**
    - apple juice – fexofenadine, atenolol, aliskiren
    - orange juice – aliskiren, atenolol, celiprolol, montelukast, fluoroquinolones, alendronate
    - pomelo juice – sildenafil
    - grape juice – cyclosporine
- **increased drug bioavailability:**
    - Seville orange juice – felodipine
    - pomelo juice – cyclosporine
    - orange juice – aluminum-containing antacids (Bailey, 2004)

Juice-drug interaction consequences are influenced by many factors like the amount consumed, fruits mixed or not with other fruits and vegetables, the time between juice drinking and drug intake, genetic polymorphism, and diverse individual factors of each person (Chen M. e., 2018). But since both preventing cancer by veganism and juicing detoxes are frequent in the no man's alternative land, healthcare professionals working in oncology settings would better ask their patients presenting unexpected or unexpectedly high side effects about such dietary practices before considering starting or stopping an essential treatment. The patient is not a passive recipient of treatment.

Professional nutrition does not sustain extreme recommendations and ping-ponging between eating just meat, eggs, cheese, and cereal or eating just veggies and fruits. Both extremes are unhealthy. Nutritional deficiencies can occur both if we go too low carb and eat just meat, dairy, eggs, and whole grains (Al-Reshed, 2023) and if we eat just veggies and fruits like in the vegan diet (Bakaloudi, 2021). And, at least in oncology settings, these have no real point as the WHO states that other than the excessive and frequent consumption of ultra-processed foods, the most important risk factors that are cumulatively involved in the apparition of cancer are: smoking, alcohol consumption, obesity, low fruit and vegetable intake, sedentariness, air pollution, and carcinogenic infections.

Fruits and vegetables are on the list for cancer prevention. However, approximately 2.2 million infection-attributable cancer cases were diagnosed worldwide in 2018 due to Helicobacter pylori, Human Papilloma Virus, hepatitis B and C, Epstein-Barr, and HIV (De Martel, 2020). Thus, to say that the fats, carbs, and fibers contained in foods don't influence health because they're not used in some equations and that the impact of smoking, alcoholism, obesity, sedentariness, pollution, and carcinogenic infections can be wiped by eating fruits and veggies is kind of like saying that based on mathematic calculations 1 plus 4 equals 14.

Nevertheless, nowadays, many don't look closely enough into popular dietary trends to understand how they actually work, and some have even started drinking alkaline water or buying expensive water alkalinization devices to replace acidosis with alkalosis. Without extreme dietary intakes we cannot become more alkaline or acidic because of the human body's pH buffering systems. Sadly this can happen in about two weeks by drinking alkaline water (Heil, 2010). And I wrote "sadly" for three reasons:

- **It's a waste of money as anyone can instantly become alkaline when they get sick:**
    o vomit (Mehler, 2016),
    o have a thermal shock in heat stress (Bain, 2011),
    o have fever (Schuchmann, 2011),
    o have a stroke (Zöllner, 2015).
- **Chronic alkalosis is detrimental as the lower gastric pH is beneficial for:**
    o The absorption of vitamin B12 and vitamin C, iron, and calcium (Carabotti, 2021).
    o Optimal pharmacokinetics of targeted anticancer medications (Budha, 2012).
    o And since we have data recommending clinicians to avoid unnecessary proton pump inhibitors prescription based on studies showing that their use in patients treated with immune checkpoint inhibitors is associated with shorter overall survival (Chen B. e., 2022), should we risk increasing gastric pH with alkaline water?
- **The target audience is often oncology patients and their caregivers.**

The attempt to counteract the extracellular acidosis that comes along with aerobic glycolysis by drinking alkaline water ignores the fact that in vivo tumors are heterogeneous and that malignant cells are highly adaptive.

While some preclinical studies performed on glycolytic cancer cellular lines show that extracellular alkalinity could contribute to destroying them (Yustisia, 2017), other preclinical studies performed on other cancer cells that don't use the aerobic glycolysis show that alkalinization helps them proliferate and metastasize (Wanandi, 2017). And even in tumors with the same breast localization, we cannot simply tell by default that drinking alkaline water associates apoptosis or malignant proliferation and metastasis, as many cancers developed by themselves in living humans are heterogeneous (Choi, 2013).

Despite the promotion of the alkaline diet and alkaline water by the lay media and the many salespeople, we have no RCTs performed on oncology patients to prove that alkaline water contributes to healing any cancer or that it prevents such diagnosis, researchers considering that promoting alkaline water is scientifically unjustified (Fenton, 2016).

And I'd like to stay a second more on the financial toxicity, which is frequently left aside.

What I can say after a decade of working in oncology is that the diagnosis and the many treatments hijack patients' minds and lives. And while most of us would be as emotionally hurt by such a dreadful situation, one of the most overlooked unwanted consequences is financial toxicity.

In the despair and confusion generated by diagnosis, especially younger patients with cancer are tempted to spend any amount of money on complementary therapies. But impulsively trying to soothe despair and confusion by buying things can have a high cost in oncology. And while financial education is desperately needed for people diagnosed with cancer, a study performed in eight countries in Asia shows that 48% of cancer patients go into a financial collapse one year after the diagnosis (ACTION Study, 2015).

Financial toxicity of cancer treatment is a global problem, with most health systems not ensuring equal access to diagnosis and treatment. In rich countries, the concept is ignored by many patients and caregivers during active oncology treatment, especially when health insurances cover the cost of the treatment. And, if the state pays for the allopath treatment, the patient and caregivers seem eager to pay out of their own pocket like there's no tomorrow, although we know that 35% of patients living in rich countries risk medical-related impoverishment, the percentage increasing to 79% in low- and middle-income countries (Ehsan, 2023).

In other countries than the rich ones, the patient must cover more than half of the cost of the treatment and follow-up. This does not consider the housing and food costs of the patient who is no longer working, thus spending from a waning financial resource to which only the rest of the family members can contribute (Bhoo-Pathy, 2019). And while, for instance, returning to work after a breast cancer diagnosis is a marker of psychosocial return to the life before the disease in reality things don't always go as expected.

Fatigue, memory and cognition disturbances, stress, pain, hot flushes, lymphedema, paresthesia, sleep disturbances, depression, anxiety, and sometimes the unaddressed shame generated by the new body image changes are factors that can decrease patients' capacity to work. Additionally, in the harsh worldwide economy post-pandemic, the return to work may involve factors like regional job availability and racial discrimination (Emerson, 2023).

A cancer diagnosis alone is frequently insufficient to motivate people to change their diet (Aldossari, 2023). And many patients try to buy the benefits any other way instead of making an effort to change their diet, which sometimes feels like such a pointless hassle.

While paying the price for all sorts of shortcuts seems justified because it makes the patient feel emotionally better, it is important to acknowledge upfront and purposefully keep in mind—as an oncology treatment access strategy—that this coping behavior can add up to a financial disaster.

Chapter 11

Intermittent fasting

Since the Japanese cell biologist Yoshinori Ohsumi was awarded the Nobel Prize in Physiology in 2016 for his preclinical data showing how starved cells adapt by recycling their content through autophagy, more and more people have been drawn to intermittent fasting as a more user-friendly way to mimic starvation, some to prevent cancer, some to lose weight, and some to stay young.

In English, "auto" means "self," and "phagy" means "eat;" thus, the verbatim meaning of "autophagy" is "self-eating." The number of people subscribing to the idea that they might get health, beauty, and youth by not eating—in order to self-eat—is growing every day.

Many seem to forget that the only cells able to not grow old and die as they're naturally supposed to are the cancerous cells. And even though the scientific evidence on fasting-induced autophagy and its' rejuvenation benefits is barely there as a preclinical concept, the joint venture between the weight loss, the anti-cancer, and the youth-vending industries are selling the embryo before becoming a baby. And buyers are many.

There is zero human data showing an anti-tumor effect for fasting-induced autophagy.

Autophagy may lower cancer risk, but all we have is Janus-faced preclinical data (Debnath, 2023).

The hope is kept alive by preclinical studies suggesting that several cancerous cell lines can be removed by autophagy (Galluzzi, 2015).

However, the available preclinical data is far more complicated than the straightforward assumption implied by the growing fasting community, showing that although the natural autophagy process does decline with age, potentially allowing damaged cells to multiply and grow into tumors, cells that already became neoplastic can use autophagy as an adaptive way to overcome metabolic distress, hence favoring treatment resistance (Wu W. K., 2012).

Nonetheless, many are beaming with confidence, ignoring autophagy's ability to both inhibit tumorigenesis plus promote cancer progression and drug resistance (Qin Y. e., 2023), while the clinicians who ignore that the current evidence is merely preliminary jump the gun (Wu Q. a., 2023) recommending starvation to cancer patients because "some clinical studies suggest that intermittent fasting may improve fatigue and reduce gastrointestinal toxicities in certain patients with cancer" (Sucholeiki, 2024).

Despite the hope, fasting has no proven beneficial effect on reducing side effects and toxicities in oncology (Drexler, 2023).

And although the high enthusiasm of the clinicians eager to recommend intermittent fasting based on preclinical data during harsh chemotherapy and radiotherapy regimens seems unbelievable from a professional nutrition standpoint, what's even more unbelievable is when surgeons recommend fasting too, forgetting all the decades of enhanced recovery after surgery (ERAS) research that promote minimal preoperative fasting.

The main reason why minimal fasting before surgery was recommended in the first place within the ERAS protocol was to reduce the postoperative insulin resistance and cortisol levels as much as possible by preoperative carbohydrate loading (Ackerman, 2020).

However, in the obesity epidemics we all witness today worldwide, many have no recollection that insulin resistance is a protective mechanism that also happens after fasting, not only after overeating (Soeters, 2012). And when this is coupled with a popular dietary trend, what we all witness is fatter and fatter patients with temporarily smaller bodies until the long-term disturbed eating behavior and obesity visibly show up to party (Dulloo & Montani., 2015).

ERAS sustains the early return to normal life by significantly reducing opioid use and length of hospital stay and by minimal preoperative fasting followed by resuming normal eating during the day of the operation, all these without increasing complication or readmission rates. However, although ERAS protocols have gained conceptual acceptance by many surgical specialties, the clinical practice introduction of a new protocol as complex as ERAS can take a long time. In many clinical settings, the implementation is either refused from the get-go or incomplete due to all sorts of resource-related, staff-related, or patient-related issues (Offodile, 2019).

At conferences, many speak highly of ERAS. But even the people presenting stuff at conferences may act differently in their clinical practice. In reality, more than two decades after the introduction of the 2h liquid carbohydrate loading limit, many patients are still recommended to fast for a median of up to 12h before anesthesia, mainly because of old inertia, rigidity, and system issues (Rüggeberg, 2024). And patients undergoing oncology surgery report the longest perioperative fasting (Beck, 2023).

Thus, although traditional preoperative fasting is truly and scientifically proven out of date, perhaps the main thing to consider when evaluating the real-world low clinical implementation of ERAS is that it is mainly done by informal learning and subjective views on the matter, medical residents learning it by imitating their seniors. When the senior surgeon doesn't agree or even consider it, the residents will mainly follow (Jogerst, 2023). Consequently, in some parts of the world ERAS is used even in patients with cardiac surgery (Kotfis, 2020) or pancreaticoduodenectomy (Noba L. e., 2023), while in the places where ERAS is not implemented patients take longer to recover even after breast surgery (Gruber, 2023).

And it is true that besides patient-related factors, the surgeon's expertise and the chosen surgical technique influence surgical outcomes. It is also true that the ERAS protocol involves many specialties that sometimes don't seem to see eye to eye in real clinical practice, a consensus review of optimal perioperative care in breast reconstruction surgery underlining as key recommendations:

- opioid-sparing perioperative medications,
- minimal preoperative fasting and early feeding,
- use of anesthetic techniques that decrease postoperative nausea, vomiting, and pain,
- use of measures to prevent intraoperative hypothermia,
- support of early mobilization after surgery (Temple-Oberle, 2017).

And as opposed to the lowered food intake over the course of the whole day classically recommended for weight loss, intermittent fasting involves only part-time restrictions: time-restricted eating, alternate day fasting, only five days a week restrictions, or intermittent energy restriction.

The many hoping that they can get their whole salary by working part-time are encouraged by the tens of reviews made on the abundant but low-quality evidence performed on mixed healthy and metabolically unhealthy people—the main message of a review of 48 systematic reviews on the highly heterogeneous intermittent fasting data suggests that the easiness to restrain oneself only for some of the time may be at least as efficient as making an effort to eat less all of the time (Lange, 2024).

People who look for quick solutions to complex problems like obesity are willing to do whatever it takes to get rid of the problem's consequences, except to deal with the root cause of the problem. As Simon Sinek would say, to find the root cause of the problem, maybe it would be wise to *Start with why*.

So, why do we eat?

To make a long story short, we eat for three reasons:

- Hunger
- Appetite
- Nothing

Hunger is a physical need for nutrients.

- It is a somatic sensation precisely located in the middle upper abdominal gastric area (Cannon W. B., 1912), with degrees of intensity (Carlson, 1913).
- It is satisfied with the feeling of satisfaction and relaxation (Monello, 1967).
- It mainly involves the hormones glucagon (Stunkard, 1955) and insulin (Rodin, 1985).

Appetite is a mental need for gratification.

- It has no physical localization, is mainly induced by food palatability (Yeomans, 2004), and feels paradoxically urgent in people with a dieting history (Bossert-Zaudig, 1991).
- It is satisfied with the feeling of fullness (Murray, 2009).
- It mainly involves the hormones leptin (Friedman, 2016) and ghrelin (Kojima, 2002), besides cholecystokinin (Degen, 2001), peptide YY (Batterham R. L., 2003), pancreatic polypeptide (Batterham R. L., 2003), glucagon-like peptide-1 (Flint, 2001), and oxyntomodulin (Cohen, 2003).

Eating for nothing is an emotional need for anesthesia.

Many people eat to numb themselves out, emotional anesthesia being obtained from the joint effects on hunger and appetite of dopamine (Wang G.-J. N., 2002), oxytocin (Leng, 2008), vasopressin (Richter C. P., 1941), serotonin (de Matos Feijó, 2011), GABA (Joshi, 2022), and cortisol (Lawson, 2011). This is generically called "emotional eating," but it is quite a complex issue covering a vast area of disordered eating behaviors more apparent in people with high negative urgency (highly impulsive behavior in response to negative emotions): binge eating, night eating syndrome, selective food craving, and compulsive or non-compulsive grazing (Heriseanu, 2017).

When life gets hard, people with lower internal power just want a break from it all. Thus some drink, some smoke, some take drugs, some buy things, some watch porn, some play video games. Others overeat. Besides the fact that it doesn't address any of the eating behavioral patterns that might have led to weight gain in the first place, the main problem with using intermittent fasting for weight loss is that it can maintain or amplify the need to eat for nothing.

Yo-yo dieting, or weight cycling, is weight loss followed by subsequent regain of the lost weight. And while nowadays it seems that a bottle of pink paint spilled over the abundant intermittent fasting literature, Islamic fasting during Ramadan remains proof of the yo-yo effect associated with time-restricted eating. Despite the high enthusiasm, a median of only 1 kg weight loss is reported at the end of Ramadan (Jahrami, 2020), and this usually lasts for about two weeks after Ramadan (Sadeghirad, 2014). Moreover, this is a median value, not the rule. A pilot study performed by 173 nutrition students on their Saudi families shows that many people gain weight although they refrain from eating during the day, reporting an increased night intake of foods rich in fat and carbohydrates and less physical exercise during the month of Ramadan (Bakhotmah, 2011).

There is one fundamental but frequently overlooked reason behind the yo-yo impact of intermittent fasting restrictions, including during and after Ramadan: the social impact of eating. Although eating remains one of the pleasurable social behaviors—as most people enjoy sharing it with each other—because of the bad publicity obesity has these days, many people went from one extreme to another, penduling from restrained eating to compulsively overeating (de Ridder, 2022). Consequently, many overeat at night during the month of Ramadan and then overeat some more during the Eid holiday at the end of Ramadan because of the abundance of delicious food shared with friends and family. And this is not about the "Ramadan fasting yo-yo effect" but about the fact that humans are herd animals.

This pendulum effect behind yo-yo dieting is masterfully portrayed in one of the many studies described in Prof. Dan Ariely's book *A Beginner's Guide to Irrational Behavior*.

People walking out of a supermarket after buying their weekly groceries were asked by his students if they were willing to donate money for poor children, and if so, how much?

And those who bought foods they perceived as unhealthy were much more willing to help the poor, unlike the ones who bought broccoli. The paradox of moral self-regulation states that acting right may lead people with low self-control to feel licensed to act badly until their built-up moral image gets threatened. Then, good behavior may be used again to repair some of the perceptual damage (Sachdeva, 2009).

And while scientists and clinicians keep on switching from authoritarian scolding to reassurance that repeated weight loss/weight regain is not that detrimental, the number of obese people is growing worldwide (Jelaković, 2023).

One billion people are obese globally because the only diet that works long-term is a true lifestyle change (Evert, 2017), and this cannot be achieved without encouraging self-management (Franklin, 2018). Although for the better part of the past century, we saw time and again that whips don't work for long-term eating behavior change, the fact that the old proposed dietary restrictions might actually be the cause of the obesity remains hard to swallow (Monnier, 2021).

Nevertheless, a cross-sectional survey performed in the US shows that 74.6% of adults have intentionally tried to lose weight, with the average number of yo-yo dieting over their lifetime being 7.82, associating internalized weight stigma which is frequently amplified by the more domineering healthcare providers (Quinn, 2020).

However, if eating for nothing is not fixed professionally by highly trained clinical psychologists, both weight regain and substance use disorders can happen even after bariatric surgery (Saules, 2018). Thus, "eat less" doesn't work for people who are emotional eaters even when surgically forced (Athanasiadis, 2021).

It is difficult to exit weight cycling and the many self-imposed dietary restraints previously used for forced weight control when weight stigma and social pressure remain on the table (Romo, 2024). And starving oneself to lose weight only increases the emotional need to overeat to numb the distress or to splurge out from time to time.

In professional nutrition practice, this behavior is called the "What the Hell!" effect, and it means to agree to abandon eating self-control because today it is… [please fill in the blank yourself: Christmas, your in-law's visit, the summer all-inclusive holiday, the neighbors' barbeque, a day where you're bored or a day where you had a fight with your significant other…].

And tomorrow will be a fresh new start.

The problem is that tomorrow can hardly be a fresh new start, specifically due to the metabolic adaptations the body uses to survive today's Hell:

- **If tomorrow, you continue to overeat**, especially high-fat foods, your body will further lower your muscle insulin sensitivity and your metabolism, consequently increasing your weight gain tendency (Parry, 2017).
- **If tomorrow, you eat too little**, your body may adapt by further lowering your muscle insulin sensitivity (Clayton, 2018) and by altering the sensitivity to the neuro-endocrine regulation of appetite, further increasing the drive to have yet another "What the Hell!" episode (O'Connor, 2016).
- **If tomorrow, you eat enough to get into energy balance and do resistance exercises**, you may increase yesterday's decreased muscle insulin sensitivity back to normal (Koopman R. e., 2005) and somehow dim down your appetite (Hägele, 2019).

No diet alone can fix the metabolic damage done by a "What the Hell!" episode (Ding C. e., 2019), this seemingly free license to eat being one of the most important behavioral causes of obesity.

And neither can sports alone, as even brief and modest overeating can impair insulin sensitivity and upregulate the genes involved in increased abdominal adiposity, the same in exercisers as in sedentary people (Ludzki, 2022). And although aerobic activities like running or fast walking remain alternatives to resistance training, their intensity has to be high enough to elicit metabolic adaptations, as the popular strategy to do low-intensity cardio for longer to burn more calories remains less efficient in fixing the lowered insulin sensitivity (Ortega, 2015).

Nonetheless, it is also important to keep in mind that many people who emotionally eat may also binge on sports activities in the attempt to wipe away their overeating episode's consequences, the dysfunctional exercising being a symptom of eating disorders that precedes, maintains and exacerbates the pathology (Quesnel, 2023). And because many are encouraged to fix a "What the Hell!" episode with fasting, the metabolic damage increases over time, becoming harder and harder to fix.

Each time you mentally accept to fall for it, you get more stuck on the dieting/eating-for-nothing roller-coaster. Time-restricted eating recognizes or fixes none of that. And while the intermittent restriction looks built in the very word's definition, numbing out by eating pretty much negates any attempt to lose weight, having a snowball effect even when only little amounts of foods are consumed as uninhibited grazing in response to distress (Teodoro, 2021).

Moreover, restricting eating too far to accelerate weight loss may put gas on the emotional fire.

Thus before combining energy restriction with time-restricted eating strategies "to get more or faster results" we need to remember that the available literature shows that these are mostly short-term, while the biology of human starvation was left on the table a long time ago, ever since the study performed shortly after the second world war by the very same Ancel Keys, who a decade later revolutionized the world by recommending margarine instead of butter when he invented the first "Mediterranean" diet (Keys A. e., 1950).

The Minnesota Starvation Experiment was a laborious study performed to understand the impact of the chronic undernourishment experienced during the war and to find adequate solutions to refeed the previously starved people thereafter. The experiment was conducted in 4 stages:

- **The first three months were the control period**: researchers collected data on study participants' normal eating behaviors and then provided all the required food by a full-time cook under the supervision of a trained dietitian. Each individual's meals were calculated to fit their body size in order to maintain energy balance. They consumed around 3500 calories per day, with an appropriate amount of macro- and micronutrients.
- **The next six months were the semi-starvation period**: participants were served only two meals a day, being restricted to 1570 calories a day to mimic the war conditions. As a result:
  o participants' weight dropped by 25% and their muscle mass dropped by 40%,
  o many experienced anemia, fatigue, apathy, weakness, irritability, neurological deficits, lower extremity edema, gastrointestinal discomfort, dizziness, headaches, cold intolerance, and hair loss.

- **The last three months were the controlled recovery period**: participants were divided into four groups refed with different caloric amounts.
- **An additional two months of unrestricted rehabilitation was held for 12 people.** During the first two weeks of this unrestricted period, each participant was allowed to choose their own meals, and many went as high as 7000-10000 calories per day.

The big fat surprise was not that participants' bodies changed during the study but that the prescribed and freely accepted semi-starvation had a long-term detrimental impact on their psychological well-being. Compared to the start of the study, during the semi-starvation stage, participants exhibited:

- intense preoccupation with food at such a high level that it inflicted their ability to focus,
- increased possessiveness over their food, guarding it with their elbows while worrying that others may try to eat their meals,
- lowered satiety perception, participants being recorded "licking" their plates clean,
- increased negative effect toward food being wasted, participants becoming upset by watching study non-participants in the cafeteria who didn't eat everything on their plates,
- compensatory hand-to-mouth behaviors to self-soothe feeling hungry:
  o those who used gum started chewing to excess; participants quickly chewed 2-3 sticks of gum at a time so frequently and to such an extent that their mouths became sore, and researchers had to restrict the permitted amount of gum packages to two per day,
  o those who used to smoke smoked even more to get some relief from hunger.

Using the Minnesota Multiphasic Personality Inventory, researchers logged significant increases in the hysteria, hypochondria, and depression scales, which confirmed the observed increased anxiety related to bodily concerns and high emotional distress. However, while these seemed somehow aligned with the undernourishment period, the psychological impact was unexpectedly long-lasting, remaining present years after the study.

During the controlled starvation recovery stage, participants developed even more disordered eating behaviors:

- eating "several" meals in one sitting and developing gastrointestinal issues and headaches,
- having difficulties in perceiving satiety,
- feeling hungrier frequently throughout the day,
- developing even more anxiety and depressive symptoms, and
- binge eating in an attempt to cope with their negative emotional state and then purging to control their body image concerns.

At the beginning of the study, these men were healthy both physically and psychologically.

They freely applied to participate, and no one forced them to starve in any way.

They chose to do it pretty much like many of those freely choosing to starve themselves today.

By the end of the study, they developed symptoms similar to those of anorexia nervosa, bulimia, and binge-eating disorder—an intense focus on eating that hijacked their lives.

And what was the most striking was that these healthy young men who had been mostly extroverted in their social life before participating in this two meals-a-day, semi-starvation study became isolated, felt socially inadequate, and reported a decrease in their sex drive.

And those who cannot remember the past are doomed to repeat it.

As long as eating for nothing remains on a table where a psychologist doesn't eat, any obtained weight loss is short-lived and modest, and the long-term efficacy of interventions performed in people with emotional disorders, eating remains low (Cuzzolaro, 2015). And if reading the past century's data on the human body's adaptation to starvation might not be that appealing, we could replace a thousand debates on the current trend of intermittent fasting by watching the movie *Cinderella Man*.

Chapter 12

Ketogenic diet

According to the old Byzantine fault, once upon a time, two generals wanted to conquer a highly fortified city. Today, the oncology multidisciplinary team wants to conquer cancer. Then and now, the only chance to win is a synchronized attack, and in day-to-day clinical practice, traitors arise. The first traitor seems to be obesity because it increases the risk of developing many cancers. So, nutritionists worldwide gathered their forces to boldly go where no one had gone before and "Just do it!" Consequently, a myriad of diets and dietary supplements were developed to help those in need (Murphy J. L., 2021). The second traitor—many miss when analyzing some of the obesity, cancer, or obesity & cancer defeats they stumbled upon in their lives—is the Dunning Kruger effect.

When we're new to a field, the little information we just came across seems all we need to know. And the less we know about something, the more confident we are that we know all there is to know. This is a double-edged sword as while it seems to make our lives easier, using it to cut through entire professional fields outside of our area of expertise can lead to identity-ingrained misbeliefs and poor clinical outcomes.

And without sufficient awareness and respect for the other professions, this can be any of us.

In academic settings, I could talk confidently about why I'm against axillary dissection in young women with axillary micromets after neoadjuvant chemotherapy in luminal A, lobular breast cancer.

However, this gets completely different in clinical settings, as professional wisdom involves not only academic facts gathered in trials but also the ability to recognize when a knowledge limit has been reached. And although I think I could literally debate God on the use of chemotherapy in young women with advanced luminal lobular breast cancers with positive axilla upfront, the truth is that there is currently insufficient scientific data to back up this clinical conclusion. There is no proof to show that chemotherapy is useful in such cases either—this being an extrapolation from the available ductal data as overall survival benefit is barely there even for the rare, atypical ER−/HER2+, ER+/HER2+, or triple-negative lobular breast cancers.

While I usually ask a million questions, and while I try my best to keep up to date with the many different oncology treatments, and while I can talk at nauseam about the things I don't understand with the colleagues I consider well-trained enough to explain the things I don't understand, when faced with such a situation in clinical practice at most I suggest that the patient asks for a second opinion from a professional within that specific area of expertise as I clearly acknowledge that outside my field I may not recognize when a knowledge limit has been reached and what to do about it.

Professional lines seem to become somewhat blurry when it comes to nutrition, though many healthcare providers with zero professional nutritional training feel by default equipped to extrapolate their expertise and advise the patient to do this or that based on things they witnessed in an unprofessional course they took, or on popular things they read or heard about.

The unaddressed high rates of malnutrition existent even in the most highly rated hospitals worldwide, the increased non-communicative diseases incidence, and the more than 2.5 billion people overweight and obese worldwide might beg to differ.[15] Irrespective, this derisive attitude toward professional nutrition has been on the table for decades (le Riche, 1981).

And maybe because they refuse to acknowledge that nutrition is a behavioral science, or maybe because they don't understand how much they don't know about the many things influencing eating behavior, for the past years, more and more clinicians have started to recommend ketogenic diet in oncology settings because—apparently—there's a lot of science behind it, and because—supposedly—cancer cells are dependent on aerobic glycolysis to survive; thus decreasing carbohydrate intake might also be a beneficial metabolic treatment for cancer. Thus, please take a moment to acknowledge:

What do you know about ketogenic diets in oncology settings? Would you like to help your patients with an additional cancer metabolic treatment too? Are you enticed by the rapid weight loss and hope that ketogenic diets can kill two birds with one stone?

The first thing to know in oncology is that ketogenic diets are not high-protein diets.

If you're like most people, you equal low carb with ketogenic. And many baptize "ketogenic" whatever low-carb diet they may invent these days. This makes the evaluation of the current ketogenic literature difficult as data is mixed just enough to keep up the faith that if one would somehow muster the force to "Just do it!" ketosis will be there to save the day.

---

[15] https://www.who.int/news-room/fact-sheets/detail/obesity-and-overweight

Despite the excitement, most of the current data has such a high risk of bias that the evidence for all proposed outcomes is low to very low certainty, even for drug-resistant epilepsy (Martin-McGill, 2020).

The term ketogenic implies a diet that induces increased levels of circulating ketone bodies that should be measured in blood (beta-hydroxybutyrate), urine (acetoacetate), or breath (acetone) to attest to the ketogenic metabolic condition. However, most of the available studies have measured none of these (Szendi, 2024). In clinical practice, the use of these loosely defined dietary strategies is not evidence-based and different healthcare providers decide to recommend whatever they subjectively label "ketogenic." Nevertheless, like how the Hans Krebs Nazi general sounds kind of the same as the Hans Krebs scientist, so are the two different types of low-carb diets:

- Low-carb high-fat diet
- Low-carb high-protein diet

Classic ketogenic diets were defined by the high-fat/low-carbohydrate ratio since the early 1920s, <u>with zero consideration for protein intake</u> as this was decreased to as low as 5-10% (Wilder R, 1922). And today, the protein intake in most versions of the "modified ketogenic" diets tops 20%, which is pretty much the same 0.8g/kg/day recommended to the general population outside oncology settings. This alone is enough to take them out of oncology settings as cancer patients require a higher protein intake than the general population, with guidelines endorsing a protein intake of up to 1.5 g/kg/day during all stages of active oncology treatments (Muscaritoli M. e., 2021). But since most people talking to oncology patients about what they presumably should or should not eat are not oncology nutrition professionals, let's continue the saga.

The ketogenic diet was developed in the 1920s by Russell Wilder at the Mayo Clinic based on his observations that such diets had an anticonvulsant effect in children with refractory epilepsy (Wilder, 1921). He proposed a 4:1 fat-to-carbohydrate ratio, mainly of long-chain, saturated fatty acids. The diet was hard to implement in pediatric neurology clinical practice due to gastrointestinal disturbances, hyperlipidemia, hyperuricemia, lethargy, infectious diseases, and hypoproteinemia. Data show that patients prescribed therapeutic ketogenic diets need to be monitored for osteopenia, nephrolithiasis, right ventricular diastolic dysfunction, and growth retardation.

The total retention rates of the diet in pediatric neurology—where children are kind of forced to do it as a last resort by increasingly scared and desperate parents—are 45.7% at one year and 29.2% at two years. However, even in such a case, the most important thing underlined by the data is that the diet is frequently stopped due to a lack of efficacy (Cai, 2017). Therefore, with the introduction of anticonvulsant medication, the ketogenic enthusiasm dimed off for a while.

The diet was brought back to the public attention in the 1970s by Atkins, who promoted its rapid weight loss-associated effects (Atkins, 1972). Then it fell back aside again due to the short-lived weight loss followed by the fast weight regain.

Nowadays, it got way back up. And although the up-and-down 100-year history of the ketogenic diet could be enough of a concern for those trying to keep their patients as metabolically stable as possible, as is usually the case in oncology, many healthcare providers started to consider it in clinical practice, ignoring the missing long-term safety data.

In the short-term, it all seems as rosy as Nazism might have felt initially to the non-Jewish Germans.

The rapid weight loss many enjoy initially happens by dehydration, based on the fact that the low carbohydrate intake generates glycogenolysis, 3g of water being lost for each g of the ± 500g of glycogen available in an adult human body (Flatt J., 1995). Thus, most of the fast initial weight that is lost does not come from fat but from the glycogen depletion-associated water loss. Consequently, depleting glycogen stores means you can drop 1–2 kg quickly in a couple of days depending on how much glycogen you have stored in your body, with some people having more and some having less. This is water weight loss and—regrettably for those using ketogenic diets in the attempt to lose weight—it is regained as soon as one resumes eating carbohydrates, and glycogen stores get filled back up, 3g of water being retained with each gram of restored glycogen.

The initial weight loss may continue longer-term at a slower pace in people who eat less and less due to the gradual food disgust induced by high fat intake. But this does not happen to everyone. The few available long-term data show that although the fat intake has a satiating effect via cholecystokinin, ketone bodies seem to be able to generate the need to increase food intake (Paoli, "Ketosis, ketogenic diet and food intake control: a complex relationship.", 2015). Thus, while some people may perceive more satiety, a ketogenic diet does not necessarily lead to lower food intake. This appetite disturbance puts a deadline on the initial weight loss unless one somehow manages to eat less. And the less one eats to lose weight, the less one can eat to avoid weight regain.

The price for the impressive initial weight loss is a higher tendency to gain weight when eating less than you used to, while the appetite gets further and further disturbed. Thus, to somehow address this issue, there are currently three other major modified versions of the classic ketogenic diet: the modified Atkins diet, the medium-chain triglyceride ketogenic diet, and the low glycemic index diet.

What frequently hooks people in is the impressive glycogen depletion water weight loss. Since glycogen is also stored in the muscles, not only in the liver, athletic people with more muscle mass experience higher amounts of initial weight loss than those with lower muscle mass. This type of diet looks even more impressive in highly active men. On the other hand, many sedentary people who start the diet with low muscle mass frustratingly discover that even this strategy doesn't work for them.

This happens because there are two kinds of answers to low carb: ketosis and gluconeogenesis.

The assumption that low carb = ketogenic ignores gluconeogenesis.

And reality has this funny way of remaining real in front of assumptions.

The concept that amino acids are not used for energy is an old assumption contradicted by data showing that the higher the protein intake, the more they're used as an energy supply (Gerald, 2018). Under energy and nitrogen balance, energy is derived from amino acids in about the same proportion as protein is present in the diet. When amino acid intake is higher than what would be enough for protein synthesis, the excess can be metabolized to compounds that can enter the Krebs cycle for the production of energy in the form of ATP if there is no other energy source or if the energy requirements are higher than the ones produced from carbs and fats. Under energy depletion, though, amino acids group themselves up into two categories: ketogenic (forming acetoacetate or Acetyl-CoA) and glucogenic (forming pyruvate, α-ketoglutarate, succinyl CoA, fumarate, or oxaloacetate).

Of the 20 amino acids, only two are exclusively ketogenic: leucine and lysine.

And this is not news, as Edson, alongside the scientist Hans Krebs, showed in the 1930s that:

- only the two amino acids cited above are exclusively ketogenic,
- some amino acids are not able to be either ketogenic or glucogenic, while some are able to be both,
- most amino acids are antiketogenic, being exclusively glucogenic (Edson, 1936).

The rationale supporting the potential efficacy of the ketogenic diet in epilepsy and weight loss is built on the fact that ketones are utilized as the primary energy source, as opposed to glucose, but on a low protein intake. However, the lowered dietary carbohydrate intake per se does not necessarily induce ketosis. Although ketones have an anticonvulsant or neuroprotective effect, and although their metabolization is associated with fast weight loss, none happen unless you somehow get to ketones. And about half of the people trying to follow a ketogenic diet don't manage to get or stay there because the implied ketosis doesn't just happen simply because you went low carb.

Moreover, fat doesn't magically disappear from the human body when ketones arrive.

Fat loss happens when fatty acids are introduced into the Krebs cycle and metabolized up to ATP, CO_2, and water. This mainly happens inside the muscles, which is why the increased energy needed by sports is essential for fat loss.

Although using ketones when the going gets rough is promoted as a way to protect muscle mass to be used by any tissue for energy production, ketones must somehow be introduced back into the Krebs cycle. And this cannot happen without making oxaloacetate either from carbs or from the glucogenic amino acids. To get energy from ketones, they need to be converted back to Acetyl-CoA, and Acetyl-CoA can do zilch without oxaloacetate:

- When both carbs and proteins are low, ketones can be introduced into the Krebs cycle by making oxaloacetate from structural muscle proteins through gluconeogenesis.
- When carbs are low and proteins are high, ketones can be introduced into the Krebs cycle by making oxaloacetate from the eaten dietary proteins and/or structural muscle proteins through gluconeogenesis (Krebs H., 1960).

And if you'd bear with me a little more, each step into the ketones' metabolism can be stopped by an elevated circulating insulin level or by a deregulated insulin/glucagon ratio: the higher the hunger, the higher the glucagon, which may bring up some light into understanding ketogenic diets long-term:

- Although short-term ketogenic diets may initially lower insulin resistance, the link between ketogenic diets and diabetes gets blurred in the long-term by the fact that glucagon stimulates insulin secretion (Robertson, 2023).
- Glucagon also induces skeletal muscle insulin resistance, favoring the hepatic glycogen refill by blocking the muscles' entrance of the glucose made inside the body (Adeva-Andany, 2019).
- Any fat transported to be burned inside the muscles remains untouched inside the muscles if either physical exercise is low or if carb intake or protein intake is not high enough to maintain the oxaloacetate supply needed for ketones to be metabolized (Paoli, 2023). This further decreases muscle insulin sensitivity by the subsequent increased intramuscular fat content (Bergman, 2020).

- Both sedentariness and any little slip of the ketogenic diet puts gas on all these by amplifying glucagon secretion, causing glucagon resistance in healthy but sedentary individuals (Suppli, 2024). And—if practiced on and off—ketogenic diets may have such a negative effect on fat-free mass that it cannot be corrected even by resistance training (Ashtary-Larky, 2022).

A true ketogenic diet could be therapeutic, as ketones have an anticonvulsant effect. It could be an initial step in fighting obesity if we focus on total body weight loss alone and disregard all else that eating means for humans. However, the human data shows that the more moderate, "modified ketogenic" protocols characterized by the low carb ± 30% fat intake and moderate/high protein content are not ketogenic by themselves, potentially becoming mildly ketogenic only when a very low-caloric restriction is also applied. Without the starvation impact induced by caloric restriction, isocaloric low-carb, high-protein diets don't necessarily get to become ketogenic (Tagliabue, 2024).

Low-carb high-protein diets have a chance to improve body composition without muscle loss in physically active people who would require such a nutrition intervention, while the true low-carb high fat ketogenic diet may associate muscle and performance loss even in highly active healthy people. Whilst in sedentary people, the many modified versions labeled "ketogenic" are a ride for life on the ketosis/gluconeogenesis roller-coaster that gradually leads to lower and lower metabolism by the glucagon resistance's subsequent muscle protein loss and by the increased fat ectopically deposited inside the muscle. While if we look from the helicopter, this may still look like "muscle mass," the ectopic fat moved into the muscles is in no way healthy either in healthy adults (Nachit, 2023) or in people with cancers (Aleixo G. F., 2020).

Myosteatosis may be present in people with a normal quantity of muscle mass independent of BMI, which is why evaluating muscle quality remains essential both when it comes to obesity and when it comes to oncology (Weinberg, 2018).

These 100-year-old biochemistry lessons are confirmed by newer preclinical studies showing that for a low-carb diet to induce ketosis, it must be low in protein (Bielohuby, 2011), and by the many frustrated humans who find that although they do their best to follow what they're encouraged to call a "ketogenic" diet, they either don't develop ketosis, or they're unable to stick to it.

Ketogenic waters are muddied by the mixed data that puts [low-carb high-fat ketogenic diets] and [low-carb high-protein antiketogenic diets] under the same "ketogenic" data, based on the many subjective definitions, high bias, and flawed study design. The knowledge about the long-term effect of true ketogenic diets remaining scarce and mainly extrapolated from the available short-term data (Crosby, 2021). And besides the short-term design, the usual low number of participants is believed based on their words alone, as in many studies, ketosis is not evaluated by any objective measurement, being just declared by study design (Martin-McGill, 2020). Moreover, dietary-induced ketosis shows extreme fragility to both carbohydrate and protein intake and to physical exercise, that is why most people don't get there or don't get to stay there (Fukao, 2004).

Avoiding muscle loss is the only way to maintain any long-term metabolic health-related benefits. Nevertheless, due to the impressive and fast initial weight loss experienced by those with higher initial muscle glycogen, the tendency to recommend it as a panacea became higher and higher in the context of the current worldwide obesity epidemic. However, those able to maintain a true ketogenic diet are few, most finding it hard to follow it long-term.

Due to the inefficacy of the diet for effective seizure control, low variability of the permitted foods, side effects, difficulty in preparing ketogenic-specific meals, and the overall high cost of following such a diet on a day-to-day basis many break the diet even in neurology settings (Neri, 2024).

Another thing to consider is that the low carbohydrate intake must actually be kept very low to achieve ketosis; most versions of the ketogenic diets recommend less than 50g of carbs per day. This may potentially amplify oncology treatments' side effects by vitamin, mineral, and fiber deficiencies. Leaving aside the fat vs. amino acids substrate competition used by the liver to counteract the low carbohydrate availability, this very low carb intake required to get to ketosis practically translates to a very low intake of most fruits, legumes, whole grains, and starchy vegetables as 1 cup of baked beans, pasta or rice would be more than 50g of carbs all alone, while a baked potato or an apple would bring half of that. And although sticking to the <50g of carbs per day can be done by the book with high discipline and motivation in the short run, following a ketogenic diet long-term without dietary supplements can lead to micronutrient deficiencies as most of these come from foods higher in carbohydrates. Do dietary supplements replace a healthy diet?

The second thing to know in oncology is that there is no dietary treatment for cancer.

This would be redundant for people working in oncology. Just that as many healthcare providers don't know nutrition history, as most have forgotten their medical school first-year biochemistry, and as some don't seem to have a clue about cancer metabolic plasticity, one of the main hypotheses proposed to sustain the ketogenic diet in oncology is that malignant cells cannot metabolize ketones because of the mitochondria dysfunction initially proposed as an explanation for the Warburg effect.

The supposition is contradicted by a multitude of studies showing that most of these cells' mitochondria function as good as new, most types of cancer cells being able to metabolize both fatty acids and ketones (Koundouros, 2020). And even in cells whose mitochondria don't work that well, ketones promote mitohormesis, meaning de novo mitochondria biogenesis that works as good as new (Whitaker-Menezes, 2011). Nonetheless, people unfamiliar with cancer biochemistry keep on playing the Warburg story.

The old "cancer cell" concept is so simplistic that today it cannot even be didactic.

It is true that some malignant cells sometimes do not use their mitochondria, choosing aerobic glycolysis. However, different types of "cancer cells" are as different as any other cell. For instance, a metabolic analysis of 173 different cancer cell lines from 11 types of tissues shows the high metabolic diversity anyone working in oncology would expect from the tumoral heterogeneity observed in clinical practice when dealing with patients diagnosed with different cancers, even for the same body localization (Shorthouse, 2022). Still, the "don't eat sugar to starve cancer" mantra remains prevalent in oncology.

"Sugars" is a generic word used to collectively define extremely different sweeteners, ranging from sucrose to stevia, to erythritol, to maltodextrins, to high fructose corn syrup.

"Cancer" is a high-selling marketing buzzword abused in pseudo-oncology to promote anything from personal ideas to miracle products that collectively define a huge number of extremely different diseases.

The pseudo-oncology industry's marketing is built simplistically on the old Warburg effect, ignoring the vast complexity of tumors developed on their own in vivo.

But there is little evidence linking carbohydrate intake to the risk of breast cancer, even studies performed with the highly popular glycemic index showing:

- a relative risk of 1.06 barely suggested in some prospective cohort studies (Mullie, 2016),
- no statistically significant risk neither in the premenopausal or the overall postmenopausal cohort, with a hardly identified relative risk of 1.13 for carbohydrate intake calculated with sweat and tears only in the few postmenopausal women diagnosed with HR negative breast cancers (Schlesinger, 2017).

The popularity built on availability bias does not change the high complexity of different types of cancers' biology. As with any other cell in the entire human body, different types of cancer cells differ from one another depending on the type of tissue they come from.

And cells may differ even for the same cancer localization. In breast cancer, for instance, the luminal subtypes rely on a balance between de novo fatty acid synthesis and oxidation as sources for both biomass and energy, while receptor-negative subtypes overexpress genes involved in the utilization of exogenous fatty acids (Monaco, 2017).

Furthermore, cancer cells from the same localization may differ by gender too. Some cancer cells, like the ones within male breast cancers, rarely present the Warburg effect. While that may be because they're usually luminal and luminal breast cancers prefer the Reverse Warburg effect (Pavlides, 2009), almost 1000 genes were found differentially expressed between female and male breast cancers, modulating key biological processes ranging from energy metabolism to the immune system response (Callari, 2011).

Additionally, cells that choose to use the Warburg effect can stop using it whenever necessary and just sit there dormant by switching back to the use of the Krebs cycle as a perfectly normal cell—metabolic pathway called the Crabtree effect (Smolková, 2010). Other cancer cells can feed on alive nearby cells—be they benign or malignant (Kroemer, 2014)—this being other aggressive metabolic pathways called entosis or cannibalism, also found in the more resistant cancers with autophagy areas (Dziuba, 2023).

Many other types of cancer cells default to increased lipid metabolism from the get-go, such as:

- EGFR Non-Small-Cell Lung cancer (Eltayeb, 2022)
- BRAF+ melanoma (Turner, 2022)
- bladder cancer (Xiao, 2022)
- high-grade ovarian serous cancers (Braicu, 2017)
- pancreatic cancer (Swierczynski, 2014)
- HER2+ breast cancers (Ligorio, 2021)

The hypothesis that the ketogenic diet has a positive impact in oncology is built on a few low-quality, biased clinical studies with small study cohorts, heterogenous study designs, and noncomparable regimens, that show no conclusive evidence for anti-tumor effects (Römer, 2021).

Because of the vast heterogeneity of the clinical trials on what were subjectively defined as "ketogenic," the many published systematic reviews' and meta-analyses' validity is highly questionable.

To date, human trials are equivocal regarding any beneficial effects of ketogenic diets in oncology (Lane, 2021). The available data on ketogenic diets in oncology settings is mainly preclinical (Weber, 2018).

And while preclinical data is not enough to be used to make clinical recommendations to patients, even preclinical data is far grayer than many expect—some showing that ketones promote tumor growth (Bonuccelli, 2010), while others that they don't (De Feyter, 2016). Available data is also showing that:

- Chemotherapy and radiotherapy resistance are metabolically sustained through oxidative phosphorylation, not through aerobic glycolysis (Uslu, 2024).
- Ketogenic diets can interact with the pharmacokinetics of antidiabetic, antiepileptic, and cardiovascular medications with high lipophilicity (Marinescu, 2024).
- Fatty acids and ketones amplify tumoral aggressivity, being the metabolic fuel for recurrence and metastasis (Aiderus, 2018) as, for instance, HER2+ breast cancers use fatty acids to resist treatment and metastasize to the brain (Ferraro, 2021).

Prescribing ketogenic diets in oncology settings based on the supposed metabolic inflexibility is not evidence-based, as definitive conclusions are hindered by the inconsistent results and by the heterogenic human trial data (Urzì, 2023).

Due to the many adaptations developed over time for malignant cells to become a tumor in a living human, cancers' metabolic waters may go deeper than the Mariana Trench of the Pacific Ocean, and we have no clinical data to professionally recommend anything besides moderation.

And how people transition from debating the adjuvant use of capecitabine or tamoxifen in a young patient diagnosed with early ER low/PR negative/HER2 negative breast cancer who didn't achieve pCR by neoadjuvant chemotherapy to advising the same patient to follow a ketogenic diet to starve "cancer" remains a mystery.

Regardless of the confidence and enthusiasm of people allowing themselves to be driven by the Dunning Kruger effect, ketogenic diets are professionally contraindicated to any cancer patient outside clinical trials. Nevertheless, the world is full of diets made up by people confidently perpetuating unproven nutrition myths. And while many think that being a "nutritionist" means inventing diets, this is a mark of unprofessionalism. Professional nutrition has nothing to do with inventing anything but with the ability to do a situational analysis to see what about the patient's eating behavior doesn't flow with the human body's physiology and with the ability to offer an eating behavior solution to fix it within the context of that particular human's life.

Food is not just food, and patients are not just patients.

Food is family time.

Patients are humans like any of us.

Food is having an ice cream with your child in the park and breaking bread with your friends. And because of the emotional and social impact of eating, we get the highest long-term adherence when we avoid extreme nutrition recommendations.

There are zero ways in which we can starve a cancer developed on its own in a living human.

No food, diet, or dietary supplement can cure cancer.

Oncology nutrition is supportive care.

INSTEAD OF CONCLUSION

Last October, my son lost his phone and installed the *Find-my* App on my phone to look for it. He had forgotten it in the car, and using *Find-my* to find it felt so useful and nice. But then, day after day, I kept receiving notifications on my phone from *Find-my* telling me that "Device M has been lost. Do you want to delete device M from your devices?" I had no idea what Device M was, so I ignored the message that kept on coming on my phone. Then we went to Lisbon for a short family holiday, having a connecting flight through München, and, believe it or not, the first 2023 snow hit the Germans so hard that the airport shut down, and all flights were canceled. We finally got to Lisbon two days later with no luggage, which literally meant spending four days in a foreign city with two tired and quite annoyed teenagers having nothing to wear or any of their usual things. As parents, we did our best; as children, they behaved as well as they could. Then, on the trip back, München got blocked again, and we had to stay there one more unplanned extra night with our nerves overwhelmed. During the long check-in queue we ultimately took for our last flight home, I felt bombarded by the *Find-my* message asking me if I wanted to delete Device M. Exhausted, I pressed "YES" and sent it to hell. And to hell, it went!

Device M was my laptop.

It was in my purse. *Find-my* just didn't find it important to mention it…

I hadn't backed up my data for the 890 days since I bought my laptop, as I've been married to an IT specialist for 19 years now, with two IT-know-it-all father's sons; thus, nothing IT-related could ever happen to me. Why on Earth would I ever back up my data?! When I finally got home and realized what had happened and that there was literally no way to get back the contents of my laptop, it was the first time in my entire life I became speechless and completely shut down.

Imagine that by the push of a button, you lose two years of your work, two years of your life!

This book was part of the lost content, and it had taken me years to gradually gather the information and peacefully write it at my own pace. It was all lost! And I felt petrified. I couldn't recover from the emotional shock for weeks. All last December, I was grieving in silence, pretty much like a zombie in the depths of despair, doing my best to build myself back by focusing on my family and work. And then, during New Year's Night, I decided to hold onto the professionals for whom I have the high regard I considered necessary to have enough power to be my accountability partners in order to somehow make myself not quit while writing it all over again.

I am a writer, this was my fifth book, and I had already written it. Thus, I assumed it would take one or maybe two months to write it again. It took me half a year.

We think we got it.

We think it will be easy.

We assume we know things just enough.

It feels like facts are pretty bendable to our subjective views.

But even when we know things more than just enough, it takes far more to actually do the work.

I had literally no idea how it would be to write a book twice. I rationally thought that my knowledge as a writer and the PhD in Oncology Nutrition with a decade of clinical practice was enough to just do it again in no time. It's so easy to assume… The wise part of me knew upfront that I needed to tend and befriend my stronger colleagues to mentally lean on during the moments that I'd want to give up. And these moments were many. Probably as many as those trying to quit smoking or to lose weight encounter on their own journeys. Like thinking from the sidelines that running a marathon and a sprint are kind of the same and easily doable since you know how to walk, knowing something and doing something are completely different things. And if this is the case when you actually know what you're doing, things can get sideways fast when we simply assume we know what there is to know outside our field, extrapolating our expert level in areas we kind of had a glimpse on. No matter how much of an expert we are in our fields, opinionating outside of our expertise is not professional.

"Mediterranean" diet is an invention.

Low-carb diets don't equal ketogenic diets.

There is no indication of fasting in oncology.

There is no contraindication to eating milk or dairy.

A free-range chicken has redder meat than any lazy pork.

Alcohol is never indicated for cardiovascular protection professionally.

There is no oncology treatment stage when fresh fruits or vegetables are contraindicated.

There is no diagnosis with the professional recommendation to completely eliminate sugar.

There is zero benefit from vitamin D in osteoporosis prevention in patients with no deficiency.

BMI is a label that helps with nothing except to classify people in the bad, the good, and the ugly. There is no proof that weight loss improves prognosis for overweight or obese breast cancer patients. And that is because weight loss doesn't equal fat loss.

I have worked for the past decade in oncology and have heard all the above confidently prescribed to patients by healthcare providers with zero formal training in oncology nutrition. These are unprofessional assumptions, lay generalizations, and subjective beliefs that have nothing to do with professional nutrition. But since nutrition seems like a children's game as we've all eaten since birth, what's there more to know?

ABBREVIATIONS

BCRL = breast cancer secondary lymphedema

DIEP = deep inferior epigastric perforator flap

EFSA = European Food Safety Authority

EPIC = European Prospective Investigation of Cancer

ER = estrogen receptor

ERAS = enhanced recovery after surgery

HER2 = human epidermal growth factor receptor 2

HR = hormone receptor

IARC = International Agency for Cancer Research

pCR = pathologic complete response

PR = progesterone receptor

RCT = randomized controlled trial

WHO = World Health Organization

REVIEWED SCIENTIFIC LITERATURE

Aapro, M. e. (2018). *"Management of anaemia and iron deficiency in patients with cancer: ESMO Clinical Practice Guidelines."*. Annals of Oncology.

Aapro, M. e. (2021). *"Practice patterns for prevention of chemotherapy-induced nausea and vomiting and antiemetic guideline adherence based on real-world prescribing data."*. The Oncologist .

Abdelhamid, A. S. (2018). *"Omega-3 fatty acids for the primary and secondary prevention of cardiovascular disease."*. Cochrane Database of Systematic Reviews.

Abraham, J. E. (2015). *"A nested cohort study of 6,248 early breast cancer patients treated in neoadjuvant and adjuvant chemotherapy trials investigating the prognostic value of chemotherapy-related toxicities."*. BMC medicine.

Acevedo, F. e. (2022). *"Obesity is associated with early recurrence on breast cancer patients that achieved pathological complete response to neoadjuvant chemotherapy."*. Scientific Reports.

Ackerman, R. S. (2020). *"How sweet is this? A review and evaluation of preoperative carbohydrate loading in the enhanced recovery after surgery model."*. Nutrition in Clinical Practice.

ACTION Study, G. (2015). *"Catastrophic health expenditure and 12-month mortality associated with cancer in Southeast Asia: results from a longitudinal study in eight countries."*. BMC medicine.

Adams, G. S. (2021). *"People systematically overlook subtractive changes."*. Nature.

Adams, S. C. (2016). *"Impact of resistance and aerobic exercise on sarcopenia and dynapenia in breast cancer patients receiving adjuvant chemotherapy: a multicenter randomized controlled trial."*. Breast cancer research and treatment.

Adeva-Andany, M. M. (2019). *"Metabolic effects of glucagon in humans."*. Journal of Clinical & Translational Endocrinology.

Agnoli, C. e. (2017). *"Biomarkers of inflammation and breast cancer risk: a case-control study nested in the EPIC-Varese cohort."*. Scientific reports.

Agnoli, C. e. (2017). *"Position paper on vegetarian diets from the working group of the Italian Society of Human Nutrition."*. Nutrition, metabolism and cardiovascular diseases.

Ahmed, A. M. (2014). *"Bioavailability of calcium, iron, and zinc in whole wheat flour."*. Wheat and rice in disease prevention and health.

Ahmed, S. e. (2018). *The effects of diet on the proportion of intramuscular fat in human muscle: a systematic review and meta-analysis.* Frontiers in Nutrition.

Ahn, H. e. (2021). *"Updated systematic review and meta-analysis on diagnostic issues and the prognostic impact of myosteatosis: a new paradigm beyond sarcopenia."*. Ageing Research Reviews.

Aiderus, A. M. (2018). *"Fatty acid oxidation is associated with proliferation and prognosis in breast and other cancers."*. Bmc Cancer.

Ainsworth, B. E. (1999). *"Accuracy of recall of occupational physical activity by questionnaire."*. Journal of clinical epidemiology.

Ajabnoor, S. M. (2021). *"Long-term effects of increasing omega-3, omega-6 and total polyunsaturated fats on inflammatory bowel disease and markers of inflammation: a systematic review and meta-analysis of randomized controlled trials."*. European Journal of Nutrition.

Albani, V. e. (2016). *"Exploring the association of dairy product intake with the fatty acids C15: 0 and C17: 0 measured from dried blood spots in a multipopulation cohort: Findings from the Food4Me study."*. Molecular nutrition & food research.

Alberti, A. D. (2009). *"The Mediterranean Adequacy Index: further confirming results of validity."*. Nutrition, Metabolism and Cardiovascular Diseases.

Aldossari, A. e. (2023). *"Do people change their eating habits after a diagnosis of cancer? A systematic review."*. Journal of Human Nutrition and Dietetics.

Aleixo, G. F. (2019). *"Muscle composition and outcomes in patients with breast cancer: meta-analysis and systematic review."*. Breast cancer research and treatment.

Aleixo, G. F. (2020). *"Myosteatosis and prognosis in cancer: systematic review and meta-analysis."*. Critical reviews in oncology/hematology.

Aleixo, G. F. (2020). *"The association of body composition parameters and adverse events in women receiving chemotherapy for early breast cancer."*. Breast Cancer Research and Treatment.

Aleixo, G. F. (2022). *"Association of sarcopenia with endocrine therapy toxicity in patients with early breast cancer."*. Breast Cancer Research and Treatment.

Aleixo, G. F. (2023). *"Association of body composition and surgical outcomes in patients with early-stage breast cancer."*. Breast Cancer Research and Treatment.

Aleixo, G. F. (2023). *Association of body composition and surgical outcomes in patients with early-stage breast cancer.* Breast Cancer Research and Treatment.

Alexander, D. D. (2009). *"Quantitative assessment of red meat or processed meat consumption and kidney cancer."*. Cancer detection and prevention.

Allam, M. F. (2016). *Breast cancer and deodorants/antiperspirants: a systematic review.* Central European journal of public health.

Allred, C. D. (2001). *"Soy diets containing varying amounts of genistein stimulate growth of estrogen-dependent (MCF-7) tumors in a dose-dependent manner."*. Cancer research.

Al-Raddadi, R. e. (2018). *"Prevalence of lifestyle practices that might affect bone health in relation to vitamin D status among female Saudi adolescents."*. Nutrition.

Al-Reshed, F. e. (2023). *"Low carbohydrate intake correlates with trends of insulin resistance and metabolic acidosis in healthy lean individuals."*. Frontiers in public health.

Amar, I. D. (2024). *"Preventing Bone Loss in Breast Cancer Patients: Designing a Personalized Clinical Pathway in a Large-Volume Research Hospital."*. Journal of Personalized Medicine.

Amare, D. E. (2020). *"Anti-cancer and other biological effects of a dietary compound 3, 3'-diindolylmethane supplementation: a systematic review of human clinical trials."*. Nutrition and Dietary Supplements.

Ambra, R. S. (2022). *"A review of the effects of olive oil-cooking on phenolic compounds."*. Molecules.

Amini, B. e. (2019). *"Approaches to assessment of muscle mass and myosteatosis on computed tomography: a systematic review."*. The Journals of Gerontology: Series A.

An, J. e. (2021). *"Chronic stress promotes breast carcinoma metastasis by accumulating myeloid-derived suppressor cells through activating β-adrenergic signaling."*. Oncoimmunology.

Anderson, J. J. (2018). *"Red and processed meat consumption and breast cancer: UK Biobank cohort study and meta-analysis."*. European journal of cancer.

Appleton, B. S. (1983). *"Effect of high and low dietary protein on the dosing and postdosing periods of aflatoxin B1-induced hepatic preneoplastic lesion development in the rat."*. Cancer research.

Araya-Quintanilla, F. e. (2020). *"Effectiveness of omega-3 fatty acid supplementation in patients with Alzheimer disease: A systematic review and meta-analysis."*. Neurología.

Arayici, M. E. (2023). *"High and low dietary fiber consumption and cancer risk: a comprehensive umbrella review with meta-meta-analysis involving meta-analyses of observational epidemiological studies."*. Critical Reviews in Food Science and Nutrition.

Arends, J. e. (2017). *"ESPEN expert group recommendations for action against cancer-related malnutrition."*. Clinical nutrition.

Arends, J. e. (2017). *"ESPEN guidelines on nutrition in cancer patients."*. Clinical nutrition.

Arimon-Pagès, E. e. (2019). *"Emotional impact and compassion fatigue in oncology nurses: Results of a multicentre study."*. European Journal of Oncology Nursing.

Arora, T. e. (2016). *"The impact of sleep debt on excess adiposity and insulin sensitivity in patients with early type 2 diabetes mellitus."*. Journal of Clinical Sleep Medicine.

Artaza-Artabe, I. e. (2016). *"The relationship between nutrition and frailty: Effects of protein intake, nutritional supplementation, vitamin D and exercise on muscle metabolism in the elderly. A systematic review."*. Maturitas.

Artene, D. V. (2018). *"Factors that influence oncology nutrition efficacy in breast cancer patients under antiestrogenic treatment."*. Annals of Oncology.

Asaad, M. e. (2023). *"Impact of Obesity on Outcomes of Prepectoral vs Subpectoral Implant-Based Breast Reconstruction."*. Aesthetic surgery journal.

Asaad, M. e. (2023). *"Impact of Obesity on Outcomes of Prepectoral vs Subpectoral Implant-Based Breast Reconstruction."*. Aesthetic surgery journal .

Ashtary-Larky, D. e. (2022). *"Effects of resistance training combined with a ketogenic diet on body composition: a systematic review and meta-analysis."*. Critical Reviews in Food Science and Nutrition.

Ashwell, M. P. (2012). *"Waist-to-height ratio is a better screening tool than waist circumference and BMI for adult cardiometabolic risk factors: systematic review and meta-analysis."*. Obesity reviews.

Aslan, H. a. (2020). *"Demographic characteristics, nutritional behaviors, and orthorexic tendencies of women with breast cancer: a case–control study."*. Eating and Weight Disorders-Studies on Anorexia, Bulimia and Obesity.

Astrup, A. e. (2021). *"Dietary saturated fats and health: are the US guidelines evidence-based?."*. Nutrients.

Astrup, A. N. (2019). *"Effects of full-fat and fermented dairy products on cardiometabolic disease: food is more than the sum of its parts."*. Advances in Nutrition.

Athanasiadis, D. I. (2021). *"Factors associated with weight regain post-bariatric surgery: a systematic review."*. Surgical endoscopy.

Atkan, F. F. (2021). *"The role of alexithymia on psychological resilience in women with breast cancer."*. European Psychiatry.

Atkins, R. C. (1972). *"Dr. Atkins' diet revolution; the high calorie way to stay thin forever."*.

Attar, A. e. (2012). *"Malnutrition is high and underestimated during chemotherapy in gastrointestinal cancer: an AGEO prospective cross-sectional multicenter study.* Nutrition and cancer.

Autier, P. e. (2017). *"Effect of vitamin D supplementation on non-skeletal disorders: a systematic review of meta-analyses and randomised trials."*. The lancet Diabetes & endocrinology.

Bach, A. e. (2006). *"The use of indexes evaluating the adherence to the Mediterranean diet in epidemiological studies: a review."*. Public health nutrition.

Baer, D. J. (2002). *"Moderate alcohol consumption lowers risk factors for cardiovascular disease in postmenopausal women fed a controlled diet."*. The American journal of clinical nutrition.

Bagnardi, V. e. (2015). *"Alcohol consumption and site-specific cancer risk: a comprehensive dose–response meta-analysis."*. British journal of cancer .

Bailey, D. G. (2004). *"Grapefruit juice-drug interactions. 1998."*. British journal of clinical pharmacology.

Bain, A. R. (2011). *"Cerebral vascular control and metabolism in heat stress."*. Comprehensive Physiology.

Bajaj, M. (2012). *"Nicotine and insulin resistance: when the smoke clears."*. Diabetes.

Bajic, J. E. (2018). *"From the bottom-up: chemotherapy and gut-brain axis dysregulation."*. Frontiers in Behavioral Neuroscience.

Bakaloudi, D. R. (2021). *"Intake and adequacy of the vegan diet. A systematic review of the evidence."*. Clinical nutrition.

Bakaloudi, D. R. (2021). *"Intake and adequacy of the vegan diet. A systematic review of the evidence."*. Clinical nutrition.

Bakhotmah, B. A. (2011). *"The puzzle of self-reported weight gain in a month of fasting (Ramadan) among a cohort of Saudi families in Jeddah, Western Saudi Arabia."*. Nutrition journal.

Bali, A. a. (2023). *"The impact of a vegan diet on many aspects of health: the overlooked side of veganism."*. Cureus.

Barateiro, A. I. (2017). *"Leptin resistance and the neuro-adipose connection."*. Frontiers in endocrinology.

Barber, J. G. (1994). *Social work with addictions.* NY: New York University Press.

Barbosa, H. C. (2021). *"Empowerment-oriented strategies to identify behavior change in patients with chronic diseases: an integrative review of the literature.".* Patient education and counseling.

Barclay, N. L. (2013). *"Quantitative genetic research on sleep: a review of normal sleep, sleep disturbances and associated emotional, behavioural, and health-related difficulties.".* Sleep medicine reviews.

Barlow, I. U. (2024). *"Orthorexia nervosa versus healthy orthorexia: Anxiety, perfectionism, and mindfulness as risk and preventative factors of distress.".* European Eating Disorders Review.

Barone, I. e. (2022). *"Obesity and endocrine therapy resistance in breast cancer: Mechanistic insights and perspectives.".* Obesity Reviews.

Batterham, R. L. (2003). *"Pancreatic polypeptide reduces appetite and food intake in humans.".* The Journal of Clinical Endocrinology & Metabolism.

Batterham, R. L. (2003). *The gut hormone peptide YY regulates appetite.".* Annals of the New York Academy of Sciences.

Baudic, S. e. (2016). *"Effect of alexithymia and emotional repression on postsurgical pain in women with breast cancer: a prospective longitudinal 12-month study.".* The Journal of Pain.

Bauer, J. e. (2013). *"Evidence-based recommendations for optimal dietary protein intake in older people: a position paper from the PROT-AGE Study Group.".* Journal of the american Medical Directors association.

Bayon, V. e. (2014). *"Sleep debt and obesity.* Annals of medicine.

Beals, J. W. (2016). *"Anabolic sensitivity of postprandial muscle protein synthesis to the ingestion of a protein-dense food is reduced in overweight and obese young adults.".* The American journal of clinical nutrition.

Beasley, J. M. (2013). *"The role of dietary protein intake in the prevention of sarcopenia of aging.".* Nutrition in clinical practice.

Beavers, C. J. (2022). *"Cardio-oncology drug interactions: a scientific statement from the American Heart Association.".* Circulation.

Beck, M. H. (2023). *"Real-World Evidence: How Long Do Our Patients Fast?—Results from a Prospective JAGO-NOGGO-Multicenter Analysis on Perioperative Fasting in 924 Patients with Malignant and Benign Gynecological Diseases."*. Cancers.

Beckett, E. L. (2024). *"Health effects of drinking 100% juice: an umbrella review of systematic reviews with meta-analyses."*. Nutrition Reviews.

Beckwée, D. e. (2017). *"Prevalence of aromatase inhibitor-induced arthralgia in breast cancer: a systematic review and meta-analysis."*. Supportive Care in Cancer.

Behl, T. A. (2023). *"The effects of smoking on the diagnostic characteristics of metabolic syndrome: a review."*. American Journal of Lifestyle Medicine.

Behroozian, T. e. (2021). *Predictive factors associated with radiation dermatitis in breast cancer.* Cancer Treatment and Research Communications.

Bell, K. E. (2020). *"Bioelectrical Impedance Analysis Overestimates Fat-Free Mass in Breast Cancer Patients Undergoing Treatment."*. Nutrition in Clinical Practice.

Benasi, G. e. (2024). *"The effects of sustained mild sleep restriction on stress and distress among healthy adults: Findings from two randomized crossover studies."*. Sleep Medicine.

Benasi, G. e. (2024). *"The effects of sustained mild sleep restriction on stress and distress among healthy adults: Findings from two randomized crossover studies."*. Sleep Medicine.

Bendall, C. L. (2018). *"Central obesity and the Mediterranean diet: A systematic review of intervention trials."*. Critical reviews in food science and nutrition.

Bentley, G. e. (2024). *"Fear of cancer recurrence in breast cancer: A moderated serial mediation analysis of a prospective international study."*. Health Psychology.

Bergman, B. C. (2020). *"Exercise and muscle lipid content, composition, and localization: influence on muscle insulin sensitivity."*. Diabetes.

Bernstein, A. M. (2015). *"Processed and unprocessed red meat and risk of colorectal cancer: analysis by tumor location and modification by time."*. PloS one.

Bernstein, A. M. (2015). *"Processed and unprocessed red meat and risk of colorectal cancer: analysis by tumor location and modification by time."*. PloS one.

Berrazaga, I. e. (2019). *"The role of the anabolic properties of plant-versus animal-based protein sources in supporting muscle mass maintenance: a critical review."*. Nutrients.

Berrino, F. e. (2024). *"The effect of Diet on Breast Cancer recurrence: the DIANA-5 randomized trial."*. Clinical Cancer Research.

Bhatnagar, A. e. (2019). *"Water pipe (hookah) smoking and cardiovascular disease risk: a scientific statement from the American Heart Association."*. Circulation.

Bhatta, D. N. (2020). *"Association of e-cigarette use with respiratory disease among adults: a longitudinal analysis."*. American journal of preventive medicine.

Bhoo-Pathy, N. e. (2019). *"Financial toxicity after cancer in a setting with universal health coverage: a call for urgent action."*. Journal of oncology practice.

Bhoo-Pathy, N. e. (2019). *"Financial toxicity after cancer in a setting with universal health coverage: a call for urgent action."*. Journal of oncology practice.

Biddinger, K. J. (2022). *"Association of habitual alcohol intake with risk of cardiovascular disease."*. JAMA network open.

Bielecka, M. G. (2022). *"Antioxidant, antimicrobial and anticarcinogenic activities of bovine milk proteins and their hydrolysates-A review."*. International Dairy Journal.

Bielohuby, M. e. (2011). *"Induction of ketosis in rats fed low-carbohydrate, high-fat diets depends on the relative abundance of dietary fat and protein."*. American Journal of Physiology-Endocrinology and Metabolism.

Bittoun, R. M. (1991). *"Smoking in hospitalised patients."*. Addictive behaviors.

Blackburn, H. (1975). *"Contrasting professional views on atherosclerosis and coronary disease."*. New England Journal of Medicine.

Blanco, C. e. (2023). *"Approximating defense mechanisms in a national study of adults: prevalence and correlates with functioning."*. Translational Psychiatry.

Blew, R. M. (2002). *"Assessing the validity of body mass index standards in early postmenopausal women."*. Obesity research.

Bock, K. e. (2022). *"Sleep disturbance in cancer survivors with lymphedema: a scoping review."*. Supportive Care in Cancer.

Boffetta, P. a. (2006). *"Alcohol and cancer."*. The lancet oncology.

Boing, L. e. (2020). *"Effects of exercise on physical outcomes of breast cancer survivors receiving hormone therapy–a systematic review and meta-analysis."*. Maturitas.

Boldo, E. e. (2018). *"Meat intake, methods and degrees of cooking and breast cancer risk in the MCC-Spain study."*. Maturitas.

Bolland, M. J. (2018). *"Effects of vitamin D supplementation on musculoskeletal health: a systematic review, meta-analysis, and trial sequential analysis."*. The lancet Diabetes & endocrinology.

Bolzacchini, E. e. (2021). *"Risk of venous and arterial thromboembolic events in women with advanced breast cancer treated with CDK 4/6 inhibitors: a systematic review and meta-analysis."*. Thrombosis Research.

Bonder, R. a. (2022). *"Associations between food addiction and substance-use disorders: a critical overview of their overlapping patterns of consumption."*. Current Addiction Reports.

Bonder, R. a. (2022). *"Associations between food addiction and substance-use disorders: a critical overview of their overlapping patterns of consumption."*. Current Addiction Reports.

Bonuccelli, G. e. (2010). *"Ketones and lactate "fuel" tumor growth and metastasis: Evidence that epithelial cancer cells use oxidative mitochondrial metabolism."*. Cell cycle.

Bonuccelli, G. e. (2012). *"The milk protein a-casein functions as a tumor suppressor via activation of STAT1 signaling, effectively preventing breast cancer tumor growth and metastasis."*. Cell cycle.

Borrie, A. E. (2020). *"Genetic and clinical predictors of arthralgia during letrozole or anastrozole therapy in breast cancer patients."*. Breast Cancer Research and Treatment.

Bosi, A. T. (2007). *"Prevalence of orthorexia nervosa in resident medical doctors in the faculty of medicine (Ankara, Turkey)."*. Appetite.

Bossert-Zaudig, S. e. (1991). *"Hunger and appetite during visual perception of food in eating disorders."*. European psychiatry.
Botteri, E. e. (2017). *"Improved prognosis of young patients with breast cancer undergoing breast-conserving surgery."*. Journal of British Surgery.
Brüggemann, A. J. (2012). *"Abuse in health care: a concept analysis."*. Scandinavian journal of caring sciences.
Brachthäuser, M. a. (2024). *"Tobacco Dependence in Eating Disorders and Obesity."*. Handbook of Eating Disorders and Obesity. Berlin, Heidelberg: Springer Berlin Heidelberg.
Bradbury, K. E. (2014). *"Organic food consumption and the incidence of cancer in a large prospective study of women in the United Kingdom."*. British journal of cancer.
Braicu, E. I. (2017). *High-grade ovarian serous carcinoma patients exhibit profound alterations in lipid metabolism.* Oncotarget.
Brainard, J. S. (2020). *"Omega-3, omega-6, and polyunsaturated fat for cognition: systematic review and meta-analysis of randomized trials."*. Journal of the American Medical Directors Association.
Branco, M. G. (2023). *"Bioelectrical Impedance Analysis (BIA) for the assessment of body composition in oncology: a scoping review."*. Nutrients.
Breen, L. a. (2011). *"Skeletal muscle protein metabolism in the elderly: Interventions to counteract the 'anabolic resistance' of ageing."*. Nutrition & metabolism.
Brinchmann, B. C. (2023). *"Use of Swedish smokeless tobacco during pregnancy: A systematic review of pregnancy and early life health risk."*. Addiction.
Brooks, C. E. (2024). *"Radiotherapy trial quality assurance processes: a systematic review."*. The Lancet Oncology .
Brown, A. C. (2017). *"Kidney toxicity related to herbs and dietary supplements: Online table of case reports. Part 3 of 5 series."*. Food and Chemical Toxicology.
Brown, A. C. (2017). *"Liver toxicity related to herbs and dietary supplements: Online table of case reports. Part 2 of 5 series."*. Food and chemical toxicology.

Brown, J. C. (2012). *"Safety of weightlifting among women with or at risk for breast cancer–related lymphedema: musculoskeletal injuries and health care use in a weightlifting rehabilitation trial."*. The oncologist.

Brown, T. J. (2019). *"Omega-3, omega-6, and total dietary polyunsaturated fat for prevention and treatment of type 2 diabetes mellitus: systematic review and meta-analysis of randomised controlled trials."*. bmj.

Broyles, J. M. (2020). *"The effect of sarcopenia on perioperative complications in abdominally based free-flap breast reconstruction."*. Journal of surgical oncology.

Brunnlieb, C. e. (2016). *"Vasopressin increases human risky cooperative behavior."*. Proceedings of the National Academy of Sciences.

Brytek-Matera, A. A. (2020). *"Identifying the profile of orthorexic behavior and "normal" eating behavior with cluster analysis: A cross-sectional study among polish adults."*. Nutrients.

Brytek-Matera, A. e. (2020). *"The prevalence of orthorexia nervosa in polish and lebanese adults and its relationship with sociodemographic variables and bmi ranges: a cross-cultural perspective."*. Nutrients.

Buckinx, F. e. (2018). *"Pitfalls in the measurement of muscle mass: a need for a reference standard."*. Journal of cachexia, sarcopenia and muscle.

Buckland, G. a. (2015). *"The role of olive oil in disease prevention: a focus on the recent epidemiological evidence from cohort studies and dietary intervention trials."*. British Journal of Nutrition.

Buckland, G. e. (2009). *"Adherence to the Mediterranean diet and risk of coronary heart disease in the Spanish EPIC Cohort Study."*. American journal of epidemiology.

Budha, N. R. (2012). *"Drug absorption interactions between oral targeted anticancer agents and PPIs: is pH-dependent solubility the Achilles heel of targeted therapy?."*. Clinical Pharmacology & Therapeutics.

Bulut, E. A. (2017). *"Vitamin B12 deficiency might be related to sarcopenia in older adults."*. Experimental gerontology.

Burns, A. C. (2021). *"Time spent in outdoor light is associated with mood, sleep, and circadian rhythm-related outcomes: a cross-sectional and longitudinal study in over 400,000 UK Biobank participants."*. Journal of affective disorders.

Busatta, D. e. (2022). *"Orthorexia among patients with eating disorders, student dietitians and general population: a pilot study."*. Eating and Weight Disorders-Studies on Anorexia, Bulimia and Obesity.

Butterworth Jr, C. E. (1974). *"The skeleton in the hospital closet."*. Nutrition today.

Caan, B. J. (2011). *"Soy food consumption and breast cancer prognosis."*. Cancer epidemiology, biomarkers & prevention.

Caan, B. J. (2018). *"Association of muscle and adiposity measured by computed tomography with survival in patients with nonmetastatic breast cancer."*. JAMA oncology.

Caccialanza, R. e. (2020). *"Unmet needs in clinical nutrition in oncology: a multinational analysis of real-world evidence."*. Therapeutic advances in medical oncology.

Cady, B. (1997). *"Basic principles in surgical oncology."*. Archives of Surgery.

Cahir, C. e. (2015). *"Identifying the determinants of adjuvant hormonal therapy medication taking behaviour in women with stages I–III breast cancer: a systematic review and meta-analysis."*. Patient Education and Counseling.

Cai, Q.-Y. e. (2017). *"Safety and tolerability of the ketogenic diet used for the treatment of refractory childhood epilepsy: a systematic review of published prospective studies."*. World Journal of Pediatrics.

Callari, M. e. (2011). *"Gene expression analysis reveals a different transcriptomic landscape in female and male breast cancer."*. Breast cancer research and treatment.

Calvani, R. e. (2023). *"Diet for the prevention and management of sarcopenia."*. Metabolism.

Campbell, T. C. (1976). *"The effect of quantity and quality of dietary protein on drug metabolism."*. Federation Proceedings.

Campbell, T. C. (1976). *"The effect of quantity and quality of dietary protein on drug metabolism."*. Federation Proceedings.

Cancelo-Hidalgo, M. J. (2013). *"Tolerability of different oral iron supplements: a systematic review."*. Current medical research and opinion.

Cannon, W. B. (1912). *"An explanation of hunger."*. American Journal of Physiology-Legacy Content.

Cannon, W. B. (1993). *"An Explanation of Hunger 1."*. Obesity research.

Cao, A. e. (2022). *"Effect of exercise on sarcopenia among cancer survivors: a systematic review."*. Cancers.

Cao, J. e. (2024). *"Interaction between body mass index and family history of cancer on the risk of female breast cancer."*. Scientific Reports.

Cao, Y. e. (2015). *"Light to moderate intake of alcohol, drinking patterns, and risk of cancer: results from two prospective US cohort studies."*. Bmj.

Capel-Alcaraz, A. M. (2023). *"The efficacy of strength exercises for reducing the symptoms of menopause: a systematic review."*. Journal of clinical medicine.

Cappuccio, F. P. (2010). *"Quantity and quality of sleep and incidence of type 2 diabetes: a systematic review and meta-analysis."*. Diabetes care.

Carabotti, M. B. (2021). *"Common pitfalls in the management of patients with micronutrient deficiency: keep in mind the stomach."*. Nutrients.

Carlson, A. J. (1913). *"CONTRIBUTIONS TO THE PHYSIOLOGY OF THE STOMACH: V. The Influence of Stimulation of the Gastric Mucosa on the Contractions of the Empty Stomach (Hunger Contractions) in Man."*. American Journal of Physiology-Legacy Content.

Caroli, A. e. (2011). *"Invited review: dairy intake and bone health: a viewpoint from the state of the art."*. Journal of dairy science.

Carr, P. R. (2016). *"Meat subtypes and their association with colorectal cancer: Systematic review and meta-analysis."*. International journal of cancer.

Carter, C. S. (1999). *The integrative neurobiology of affiliation.* Mit Press.

Carter, C. S. (2017). *"The oxytocin–vasopressin pathway in the context of love and fear."*. Frontiers in endocrinology.
Carter, C. S.-A. (2017). *"14 the Roots of Compassion: An Evolutionary and Neurobiological Perspective."*. The Oxford handbook of compassion science.
Chae, Y.-R. e. (2024). *"Diet-induced gut dysbiosis and leaky gut syndrome."*. Journal of Microbiology and Biotechnology.
Champ, C. E. (2013). *Dietary recommendations during and after cancer treatment: consistently inconsistent?* Nutrition and cancer.
Chan, D. S. (2014). *Body mass index and survival in women with breast cancer—systematic literature review and meta-analysis of 82 follow-up studies.* Annals of oncology.
Chang, Y. e. (2020). *"Low levels of alcohol consumption, obesity, and development of fatty liver with and without evidence of advanced fibrosis."*. Hepatology.
Charen, E. a. (2020). *"Toxicity of herbs, vitamins, and supplements."*. Advances in chronic kidney disease.
Cheema, B. S. (2014). *"Safety and efficacy of progressive resistance training in breast cancer: a systematic review and meta-analysis."*. Breast cancer research and treatment.
Chen J, e. a. (1990). *"Diet, Life-Style, and Mortality in China: A Study of the Characteristics of 65 Chinese Counties"*. Oxford University Press.
Chen, B. e. (2022). *"Association of proton pump inhibitor use with survival outcomes in cancer patients treated with immune checkpoint inhibitors: a systematic review and meta-analysis."*. Therapeutic Advances in Medical Oncology.
Chen, C. L. (2011). *The impact of obesity on breast surgery complications.* Plastic and reconstructive surgery.
Chen, G. e. (2022). *"Gut microbiota dysbiosis: The potential mechanisms by which alcohol disrupts gut and brain functions."*. Frontiers in microbiology.
Chen, H. e. (2023). *"Impact of body mass index and its change on survival outcomes in patients with early breast cancer: A pooled analysis of individual-level data from BCIRG-001 and BCIRG-005 trials."*. The Breast.

Chen, H. e. (2023). *The relationship between central obesity and risk of breast cancer: a dose–response meta-analysis of 7,989,315 women.* Frontiers in Nutrition.

Chen, J. e. (2022). *"Formation of oxidation products in polar compounds of different vegetable oils during French fries deep-frying."*. Journal of Food Processing and Preservation.

Chen, J.-H. e. (2023). *"Missing puzzle pieces of time-restricted-eating (TRE) as a long-term weight-loss strategy in overweight and obese people? A systematic review and meta-analysis of randomized controlled trials."*. Critical Reviews in Food Science and Nutrition.

Chen, L. e. (2023). *"Impact of body mass index in therapeutic response for HER2 positive breast cancer treated with neoadjuvant targeted therapy: a multi-center study and meta-analysis."*. Breast Cancer.

Chen, L. M. (2019). *"Milk and yogurt intake and breast cancer risk: a meta-analysis."*. Medicine.

Chen, L.-K. e. (2014). *"Sarcopenia in Asia: consensus report of the Asian Working Group for Sarcopenia."*. Journal of the American Medical Directors Association.

Chen, M. e. (2014). *"Association between soy isoflavone intake and breast cancer risk for pre-and post-menopausal women: a meta-analysis of epidemiological studies."*. PloS one.

Chen, M. e. (2014). *"Association between soy isoflavone intake and breast cancer risk for pre-and post-menopausal women: a meta-analysis of epidemiological studies."*. PloS one.

Chen, M. e. (2018). *"Food-drug interactions precipitated by fruit juices other than grapefruit juice: An update review."*. Journal of food and drug analysis.

Chen, S. e. (2016). *"Dietary fibre intake and risk of breast cancer: a systematic review and meta-analysis of epidemiological studies."*. Oncotarget.

Chen, S. e. (2021). Annals of Oncology.

Chen, S.-T. e. (2022). *The impact of body mass index (BMI) on MRI diagnostic performance and surgical management for axillary lymph node in breast cancer.* World Journal of Surgical Oncology.

Chen, W. Y. (2011). *"Moderate alcohol consumption during adult life, drinking patterns, and breast cancer risk."*. Jama.

Chen, Y.-C. e. (2024). *"Global prevalence of Helicobacter pylori infection and incidence of gastric cancer between 1980 and 2022."*. Gastroenterology.

Cheng, L. W. (2024). *"Effects of aerobic combined with resistance exercise on cardiorespiratory fitness and cardiometabolic health in breast cancer survivors: A Systematic Review, meta-analysis and meta-regression."*. Heliyon.

Chéruel, F. M.-G. (2017). *"Effect of cigarette smoke on gustatory sensitivity, evaluation of the deficit and of the recovery time-course after smoking cessation."*. Tobacco induced diseases.

Chiang, S. N. (2023). *"Compound Effect of Hypoalbuminemia and Obesity on Complications after Autologous Breast Reconstruction."*. Plastic and reconstructive surgery.

Childs, E. a. (2010). *"Effects of acute psychosocial stress on cigarette craving and smoking."*. Nicotine & tobacco research.

Chlebowski, R. T. (2002). *Weight loss in breast cancer patient management.* Journal of clinical oncology.

Cho, K.-H. e. (2022). *"Long-term alcohol consumption caused a significant decrease in serum high-density lipoprotein (HDL)-cholesterol and apolipoprotein AI with the atherogenic changes of HDL in middle-aged Korean women."*. International Journal of Molecular Sciences.

Choi, J. e. (2013). *"Metabolic interaction between cancer cells and stromal cells according to breast cancer molecular subtype."*. Breast cancer research.

Choi, J. e. (2013). *Metabolic interaction between cancer cells and stromal cells according to breast cancer molecular subtype.* Breast cancer research.

Choudhry, D. N. (2024). *"The effect of resistance training in reducing hot flushes in post-menopausal women: A meta-analysis."*. Journal of Bodywork and Movement Therapies.

Choy, A. (1990). *"The winner's triangle."*. Transactional Analysis Journal .

Christodoulides, S. e. (2016). *"Systematic review with meta-analysis: effect of fibre supplementation on chronic idiopathic constipation in adults."*. Alimentary pharmacology & therapeutics.

Chrystoja, B. R. (2021). *"A systematic comparison of the global comparative risk assessments for alcohol."*. Addiction.

Chung, S. Y. (2021). *"Impact of radiation dose on complications among women with breast cancer who underwent breast reconstruction and post-mastectomy radiotherapy: A multi-institutional validation study."*. The Breast.

Cicchinelli, S. e. (2023). *"The impact of smoking on microbiota: a narrative review."*. Biomedicines.

Cichosz, G. H. (2020). *"The anticarcinogenic potential of milk fat."*. Annals of Agricultural and Environmental Medicine .

Clancy, C. e. (2020). *"Breast cancer patients' experiences of adherence and persistence to oral endocrine therapy: a qualitative evidence synthesis."*. European Journal of Oncology Nursing.

Clark, L. a. (2023). *"Engineered highs: Reward variability and frequency as potential prerequisites of behavioural addiction."*. Addictive Behaviors.

Clayton, D. J. (2018). *"24-h severe energy restriction impairs postprandial glycaemic control in young, lean males."*. British Journal of Nutrition.

Clinton, S. K. (2020). *"The world cancer research fund/American institute for cancer research third expert report on diet, nutrition, physical activity, and cancer: impact and future directions."*. The Journal of nutrition.

Coelho-Junior, H. J. (2022). *"Protein intake and sarcopenia in older adults: a systematic review and meta-analysis."*. International journal of environmental research and public health.

Cohen, M. A. (2003). *"Oxyntomodulin suppresses appetite and reduces food intake in humans."*. The Journal of Clinical Endocrinology & Metabolism.

Commane, D. e. (2005). *"The potential mechanisms involved in the anti-carcinogenic action of probiotics."*. Mutation Research/Fundamental and Molecular Mechanisms of Mutagenesis .

Condorelli, R. a.-L. (2018). *"Managing side effects in adjuvant endocrine therapy for breast cancer."*. Expert review of anticancer therapy.

Conner, T. S. (2017). *"Let them eat fruit! The effect of fruit and vegetable consumption on psychological well-being in young adults: A randomized controlled trial."*. PloS one.

Cooper, C. B. (2018). *"Sleep deprivation and obesity in adults: a brief narrative review."*. BMJ open sport & exercise medicine.

Copson, E. R. (2015). *Obesity and the outcome of young breast cancer patients in the UK: the POSH study.* Annals of Oncology.

Cormie, P. e. (2013). *"Neither heavy nor light load resistance exercise acutely exacerbates lymphedema in breast cancer survivor."*. Integrative cancer therapies.

Cornfield, J. e. (1959). *"Smoking and lung cancer: recent evidence and a discussion of some questions."*. Journal of the National Cancer institute.

Costa, A. R. (2014). *"Impact of breast cancer treatments on sleep disturbances–A systematic review."*. The Breast.

Costanzo, S. e. (2011). *"Wine, beer or spirit drinking in relation to fatal and non-fatal cardiovascular events: a meta-analysis."*. European journal of epidemiology.

Couderc, A.-L. e. (2023). *"Pre-therapeutic sarcopenia among cancer patients: an up-to-date meta-analysis of prevalence and predictive value during cancer treatment."*. Nutrients.

Covvey, J. R. (2019). *"Barriers and facilitators to shared decision-making in oncology: a systematic review of the literature."*. Supportive Care in Cancer.

Cox, R. C. (2016). *"A systematic review of sleep disturbance in anxiety and related disorders."*. Journal of anxiety disorders.

Crespi, B. T. (2022). *"Natura non facit Saltus: The adaptive significance of arginine vasopressin in human affect, cognition, and behavior."*. Frontiers in Behavioral Neuroscience.

Crockett, M. J. (2013). *"Serotonin modulates striatal responses to fairness and retaliation in humans."*. Journal of neuroscience.

Crosby, L. e. (2021). *"Ketogenic diets and chronic disease: weighing the benefits against the risks."*. Frontiers in nutrition.

Crowe, W. C. (2019). *"A review of the in vivo evidence investigating the role of nitrite exposure from processed meat consumption in the development of colorectal cancer."*. Nutrients.

Cui, Q. e. (2023). *"Validity of the food frequency questionnaire for adults in nutritional epidemiological studies: a systematic review and meta-analysis."*. Critical reviews in food science and nutrition.

Curry, B. A. (2015). *"Oxytocin responses after dog and cat interactions depend on pet ownership and may affect interpersonal trust."*. Human-Animal Interaction Bulletin.

Cuzzolaro, M. (2015). *"Eating disorders and obesity."* Clinical Management of Overweight and Obesity: Recommendations of the Italian Society of Obesity (SIO). Springer International Publishing.

Dai, X. E. (2022). *"Evolution of the global smoking epidemic over the past half century: strengthening the evidence base for policy action."*. Tobacco control.

Dalal, S. e. (2014). *"Association between visceral adiposity, BMI, and clinical outcomes in postmenopausal women with operable breast cancer."*. Journal of Clinical Oncology .

Davis, C. e. (2015). *"Definition of the Mediterranean diet: a literature review."*. Nutrients.

Dawber, T. R. (1966). *"The Framingham Study an epidemiological approach to coronary heart disease."*. Circulation.

Dawczynski, C. e. (2015). *"Saturated fatty acids are not off the hook."*. Nutrition, Metabolism and Cardiovascular Diseases.

De Blacam, C. e. (2012). *High body mass index and smoking predict morbidity in breast cancer surgery: a multivariate analysis of 26,988 patients from the national surgical quality improvement program database.* Annals of surgery.

De Feyter, H. M. (2016). *"A ketogenic diet increases transport and oxidation of ketone bodies in RG2 and 9L gliomas without affecting tumor growth."*. Neuro-oncology.

De Franceschi, L. e. (2017). *"Clinical management of iron deficiency anemia in adults: Systemic review on advances in diagnosis and treatment."*. European Journal of Internal Medicine.

De Gaetano, G. e. (2016). *"Effects of moderate beer consumption on health and disease: A consensus document."*. Nutrition, Metabolism and Cardiovascular Diseases.

De la Cruz Ku, G. e. (2022). *"Does breast-conserving surgery with radiotherapy have a better survival than mastectomy? A meta-analysis of more than 1,500,000 patients."*. Annals of Surgical Oncology.

De La Cruz Ku, G. e. (2023). *"The impact of body mass index on oncoplastic breast surgery: A multicenter analysis."*. Journal of Surgical Oncology.

De Martel, C. e. (2020). *"Global burden of cancer attributable to infections in 2018: a worldwide incidence analysis."*. Lancet Glob Health.

de Matos Feijó, F. M. (2011). *"Serotonin and hypothalamic control of hunger: a review."*. Revista da Associação Médica Brasileira (English Edition) .

De Oliveira e Silva, E. R. (2000). *"Alcohol consumption raises HDL cholesterol levels by increasing the transport rate of apolipoproteins AI and A-II."*. Circulation.

de Oliveira, L. M. (2018). *"Metal concentrations in traditional and herbal teas and their potential risks to human health."*. Science of the total environment.

de Oliveira, V. A. (2024). *"Consumption and supplementation of vitamin E in breast cancer risk, treatment, and outcomes: A systematic review with meta-analysis."*. Clinical Nutrition ESPEN.

de Ridder, D. a. (2022). *"How food overconsumption has hijacked our notions about eating as a pleasurable activity."*. Current opinion in psychology.

Deane, K. H. (2021). *"Omega-3 and polyunsaturated fat for prevention of depression and anxiety symptoms: systematic review and meta-analysis of randomised trials."*. The British Journal of Psychiatry.

Debnath, J. N. (2023). *"Autophagy and autophagy-related pathways in cancer."*. Nature reviews Molecular cell biology.

Degen, L. e. (2001). *"The effect of cholecystokinin in controlling appetite and food intake in humans."*. Peptides.

Demark-Wahnefried, W. e. (2001). *Changes in weight, body composition, and factors influencing energy balance among premenopausal breast cancer patients receiving adjuvant chemotherapy.* Journal of clinical oncology.

Demir, H. P. (2022). *"Orthorexia nervosa: The relationship with obsessive-compulsive symptoms and eating attitudes among individuals with and without healthcare professionals."*. Mediterranean Journal of Nutrition and Metabolism.

Dennert, G. e. (2012). *"Selenium for preventing cancer."*. Sao Paulo Medical Journal.

Derossis, A. M. (2003). *Obesity influences outcome of sentinel lymph node biopsy in early-stage breast cancer.* Journal of the American College of Surgeons.

Desmedt, C. e. (2020). *"Differential benefit of adjuvant docetaxel-based chemotherapy in patients with early breast cancer according to baseline body mass index."*. Journal of Clinical Oncology.

Deurenberg, P. M. (1998). *"Body mass index and percent body fat: a meta analysis among different ethnic groups."*. International journal of obesity.

Deutz, N. E. (2014). *"Protein intake and exercise for optimal muscle function with aging: recommendations from the ESPEN Expert Group."*. Clinical nutrition.

Di Cosimo, S. e. (2020). *"Effect of body mass index on response to neoadjuvant therapy in HER2-positive breast cancer: an exploratory analysis of the NeoALTTO trial."*. Breast Cancer Research.

Di Micco, R. e. (2024). *Tailoring treatment of luminal A and lobular breast cancer with 18F FES-PET/MRI: FESTA trial.* European Journal of Surgical Oncology.

Di Vincenzo, O. e. (2021). *"Bioelectrical impedance analysis (BIA)-derived phase angle in sarcopenia: A systematic review."*. Clinical nutrition.

Diallo, A. e. (2018). *"Red and processed meat intake and cancer risk: results from the prospective NutriNet-Santé cohort study."*. International journal of cancer.

Diaz, C. e. (2023). *"Artificially sweetened beverages and health outcomes: an umbrella review."*. Advances in Nutrition.

Diaz, C. e. (2023). *"Artificially sweetened beverages and health outcomes: an umbrella review."*. Advances in Nutrition.

Dietch, Z. C. (2015). *"Hypoalbuminemia is disproportionately associated with adverse outcomes in obese elective surgical patients."*. Surgery for Obesity and Related Diseases.

Díez-Arroyo, C. e. (2024). *"Effect of the ketogenic diet as a treatment for refractory epilepsy in children and adolescents: a systematic review of reviews."*. Nutrition Reviews.

Dijkstra, A. B. (2006). *"A match–mismatch test of a stage model of behaviour change in tobacco smoking."*. Addiction.

DiMarzio, P. e. (2018). *"Smoking and alcohol drinking effect on radiotherapy associated risk of second primary cancer and mortality among breast cancer patients."*. Cancer epidemiology.

Ding, C. e. (2019). *"Dose-dependent effects of exercise and diet on insulin sensitivity and secretion."*. Medicine & Science in Sports & Exercise.

Ding, C. M.-S. (2019). *"Oxytocin in metabolic homeostasis: implications for obesity and diabetes management."*. Obesity Reviews.

Ding, Y.-Y. e. (2017). *Body mass index and persistent pain after breast cancer surgery: findings from the women's healthy eating and living study and a meta-analysis.* Oncotarget.

Dinu, M. e. (2018). *"Mediterranean diet and multiple health outcomes: an umbrella review of meta-analyses of observational studies and randomised trials."*. European journal of clinical nutrition.

DiSipio, T. e. (2013). *Incidence of unilateral arm lymphoedema after breast cancer: a systematic review and meta-analysis.* The lancet oncology.

Dolezal, L. (2022). *"Shame anxiety, stigma and clinical encounters."*. Journal of evaluation in clinical practice.

Domaszewski, P. e. (2023). *"Comparison of the effects of six-week time-restricted eating on weight loss, body composition, and visceral fat in overweight older men and women."*. Experimental Gerontology.

Domic, J. e. (2022). *"Perspective: vegan diets for older adults? A perspective on the potential impact on muscle mass and strength."*. Adv. Nutr.

Domingo, J. L. (2017). *"Carcinogenicity of consumption of red meat and processed meat: A review of scientific news since the IARC decision."*. Food and chemical toxicology.

Dos Santos, B. S. (2021). *"Managing Common Estrogen Deprivation Side Effects in HR+ Breast Cancer: An Evidence-Based Review."*. Current Oncology Reports.

Dragvoll, I. e. (2022). *"Predictors of adherence and the role of primary non-adherence in antihormonal treatment of breast cancer."*. BMC cancer.

Draisci, S. e. (2019). *"Impact of body composition parameters on tumor response to neoadjuvant chemotherapy in operable breast cancer patients."*. Abstract Book XXI National Congress of Medical Oncology.

Drehmer, M. e. (2016). *"Total and full-fat, but not low-fat, dairy product intakes are inversely associated with metabolic syndrome in adults."*. The Journal of nutrition.

Drexler, U. e. (2023). *"Fasting during cancer treatment: a systematic review."*. Quality of Life Research.

Drouin-Chartier, J.-P. e. (2016). *"Comprehensive review of the impact of dairy foods and dairy fat on cardiometabolic risk."*. Advances in nutrition.

Du, M. e. (2012). *"Low-dose dietary genistein negates the therapeutic effect of tamoxifen in athymic nude mice."*. Carcinogenesis.

Duarte, C. e. (2021). *"Dairy versus other saturated fats source and cardiometabolic risk markers: Systematic review of randomized controlled trials."*. Critical reviews in food science and nutrition.

Duarte, D. C. (2011). *"The effect of bovine milk lactoferrin on human breast cancer cell lines."*. Journal of dairy science.

Dulloo, & Montani., A. G.-P. (2015). *"Pathways from dieting to weight regain, to obesity and to the metabolic syndrome: an overview."*. Obesity Reviews.

Dulloo, A. G. (1997). *"Human pattern of food intake and fuel-partitioning during weight recovery after starvation: a theory of autoregulation of body composition."*. Proceedings of the Nutrition Society.

Dwyer, J. T. (2018). *"Dietary supplements: regulatory challenges and research resources."*. Nutrients.

Dziuba, I. e. (2023). *Homotypic Entosis as a Potential Novel Diagnostic Marker in Breast Cancer.* International Journal of Molecular Sciences.

Edson, N. L. (1935). *"Ketogenesis-antiketogenesis: Ketogenesis from amino-acids."*. Biochemical Journal.

Edson, N. L. (1936). *"Ketogenesis-antiketogenesis: Substrate competition in liver."*. Biochemical Journal.

EFSA. (2012). *"Scientific Opinion on the substantiation of health claims related to soy isoflavones and maintenance of bone mineral density (ID 1655) and reduction of vasomotor symptoms associated with menopause (ID 1654, 1704, 2140, 3093, 3154, 3590)(further assessmen.* EFSA Journal.

EFSA. (2015). *"Risk assessment for peri-and post-menopausal women taking food supplements containing isolated isoflavones."*. Efsa Journal.

EFSA. (2015). *"Risk assessment for peri-and post-menopausal women taking food supplements containing isolated isoflavones."*. Efsa Journal .

EFSA Panel on Nutrition, N. F. (2021). *Scientific opinion on the relationship between intake of alpha-lipoic acid (thioctic acid) and the risk of insulin autoimmune syndrome.* EFSA Journal .

Ehsan, A. N. (2023). *"Financial toxicity among patients with breast cancer worldwide: a systematic review and meta-analysis."*. JAMA network Open.

Ekinci, E. e. (2018). *"Interventions to improve endocrine therapy adherence in breast cancer survivors: what is the evidence?."*. Journal of Cancer Survivorship.

ElAbd, R. e. (2022). *"Autologous versus alloplastic reconstruction for patients with obesity: a systematic review and meta-analysis."*. Aesthetic Plastic Surgery.

Eliassen, A. H. (2006). *Adult weight change and risk of postmenopausal breast cancer.* Jama.

Eliassen, F. M. (2023). *"Importance of endocrine treatment adherence and persistence in breast cancer survivorship: a systematic review."*. BMC cancer.

Eltayeb, K. e. (2022). *Reprogramming of lipid metabolism in lung cancer: An overview with focus on EGFR-Mutated non-small cell lung cancer.* Cells.

Emerson, M. A. (2023). "*Job loss, return to work, and multidimensional well-being after breast cancer treatment in working-age Black and White women.*". Journal of Cancer Survivorship.

Engel, R. W. (1952). "*The influence of dietary casein level on tumor induction with 2-acetylaminofluorene.*". Cancer Research.

Engel, S. e. (2019). "*Menstrual cycle-related fluctuations in oxytocin concentrations: a systematic review and meta-analysis.*". Frontiers in neuroendocrinology.

Eskandari, F. e. (2022). "*A mixed-method systematic review and meta-analysis of the influences of food environments and food insecurity on obesity in high-income countries.*". Food Science & Nutrition.

Espinoza-Derout, J. e. (2022). "*Electronic cigarette use and the risk of cardiovascular diseases.*". Frontiers in Cardiovascular Medicine.

Esposito, K. e. (2011). "*Mediterranean diet and weight loss: meta-analysis of randomized controlled trials.*". Metabolic syndrome and related disorders.

Evans, E. S. (2006). "*Impact of patient-specific factors, irradiated left ventricular volume, and treatment set-up errors on the development of myocardial perfusion defects after radiation therapy for left-sided breast cancer.*". International Journal of Radiation Oncology* Biology* Physics.

Evert, A. B. (2017). "*Why weight loss maintenance is difficult.*". Diabetes Spectrum.

Ewertz, M. e. (2011). *Effect of obesity on prognosis after early-stage breast cancer.* Journal of Clinical Oncology.

Ewertz, M. e. (2012). "*Obesity and risk of recurrence or death after adjuvant endocrine therapy with letrozole or tamoxifen in the breast international group 1-98 trial.*". Journal of clinical oncology.

Fagherazzi, G. e. (2015). "*Alcohol consumption and breast cancer risk subtypes in the E3N-EPIC cohort.*". European Journal of Cancer Prevention.

Fairfield, B. a. (2021). *"Gut dysbiosis as a driver in alcohol-induced liver injury."*. Jhep Reports.
Fan, X. e. (2023). *"A single-blind field intervention study of whether increased bedroom ventilation improves sleep quality."*. Science of the Total Environment.
Fang, P. e. (2013). *"High body mass index is associated with worse quality of life in breast cancer patients receiving radiotherapy."*. Breast cancer research and treatment.
Faraut, B. e. (2015). *"Napping reverses increased pain sensitivity due to sleep restriction."*. PloS one.
Farhat, Z. e. (2021). *"Types of garlic and their anticancer and antioxidant activity: A review of the epidemiologic and experimental evidence."*. European Journal of Nutrition.
Farvid, M. S. (2018). *"Consumption of red and processed meat and breast cancer incidence: A systematic review and meta-analysis of prospective studies."*. International journal of cancer.
Farvid, M. S. (2021). *"Fruit and vegetable consumption and incident breast cancer: a systematic review and meta-analysis of prospective studies."*. British journal of cancer.
Fedirko, V. e. (2013). *"Consumption of fish and meats and risk of hepatocellular carcinoma: the European Prospective Investigation into Cancer and Nutrition (EPIC)."*. Annals of oncology.
Feliciano, E. e. (2017). *"Prevalence of sarcopenia and predictors of body composition among women with early-stage breast cancer."*. Journal of Clinical Oncology.
Feliciano, E. M. (2019). *"Adipose tissue distribution and cardiovascular disease risk among breast cancer survivors."*. Journal of Clinical Oncology.
Felício de Souza Mamede, V. e. (2024). *"Waist Circumference as a Tool for Identifying Visceral Fat in Women with Non-Metastatic Breast Cancer."*. Nutrition and Cancer.
Fenton, T. R. (2016). *"Systematic review of the association between dietary acid load, alkaline water and cancer."*. BMJ open.
Fernandez-Sola, J. (2015). *"Cardiovascular risks and benefits of moderate and heavy alcohol consumption."*. Nature Reviews Cardiology.

Ferraris, R. P.-y. (2018). *"Intestinal absorption of fructose."*. Annual review of nutrition.
Ferraro, G. B. (2021). *Fatty acid synthesis is required for breast cancer brain metastasis.* Nature cancer.
Fillmore, K. M. (2006). *"Moderate alcohol use and reduced mortality risk: systematic error in prospective studies."*. Addiction Research & Theory.
Finkeldey, L. E. (2021). *"Effect of the intake of isoflavones on risk factors of breast cancer—A systematic review of randomized controlled intervention studies."*. Nutrients.
Fischer, J. P. (2013). *Impact of obesity on outcomes in breast reconstruction: analysis of 15,937 patients from the ACS-NSQIP datasets.* Journal of the American College of Surgeons.
Flatt, J. (1995). *Use and storage of carbohydrate and fat.* Am J Clin Nutr.
Flatt, S. W. (2010). *"Low to moderate alcohol intake is not associated with increased mortality after breast cancer."*. Cancer epidemiology, biomarkers & prevention.
Fletcher, P. C. (2018). *Food addiction: a valid concept?* Neuropsychopharmacology.
Flint, A. e. (2001). *"The effect of physiological levels of glucagon-like peptide-1 on appetite, gastric emptying, energy and substrate metabolism in obesity."*. International journal of obesity.
Flores, M. a. (2021). *"Chemistry, safety, and regulatory considerations in the use of nitrite and nitrate from natural origin in meat products-Invited review."*. Meat Science.
Fontes, F. e. (2017). *"The impact of breast cancer treatments on sleep quality 1 year after cancer diagnosis."*. Supportive Care in Cancer.
Ford, K. L. (2022). *The importance of protein sources to support muscle anabolism in cancer: An expert group opinion.* Clinical Nutrition.
Franklin, M. e. (2018). *"Patients' and healthcare professionals' perceptions of self-management support interactions: systematic review and qualitative synthesis."*. Chronic illness.

Franzoi, M. A. (2020). *"Computed tomography-based analyses of baseline body composition parameters and changes in breast cancer patients under treatment with CDK 4/6 inhibitors."*. Breast cancer research and treatment.

Franzoi, M. A. (2021). *"Clinical implications of body mass index in metastatic breast cancer patients treated with abemaciclib and endocrine therapy."*. Journal of the National Cancer Institute.

Frassetto, L. A. (2007). *Standardizing Terminology for Estimating the Diet-Dependent Net Acid Load to the Metabolic System1."*. The Journal of nutrition.

Freedman, L. S. (2014). *"Pooled results from 5 validation studies of dietary self-report instruments using recovery biomarkers for energy and protein intake."*. American journal of epidemiology.

Freigang, R. e. (2020). *"Misclassification of self-reported body mass index categories: a systematic review and meta-analysis."*. Deutsches Ärzteblatt International .

Frid, N. L. (2024). *"A systematic review on the association between body mass index and autologous breast reconstruction."*. Annals of Breast Surgery.

Friedman, J. (2016). *"The long road to leptin."*. The Journal of clinical investigation.

Fu, M. R. (2021). *The effects of obesity on lymphatic pain and swelling in breast cancer patients.* Biomedicines.

Fuchs, F. D. (2021). *"The effect of alcohol on blood pressure and hypertension."*. Current hypertension reports.

Fuchsman, K. (2023). *"Harvard Grant Study of Adult Development: 1938–2022."*. Journal of Psychohistory.

Fukao, T. G. (2004). *"Pathways and control of ketone body metabolism: on the fringe of lipid biochemistry."*. Prostaglandins, leukotrienes and essential fatty acids.

Fusconi, E. e. (2003). *"Relationship between plasma fatty acid composition and diet over previous years in the Italian centers of the European Prospective Investigation into Cancer and Nutrition (EPIC)."*. Tumori Journal .

Gabardi, S. K. (2007). *"A review of dietary supplement–induced renal dysfunction."*. Clinical Journal of the American Society of Nephrology.

Gabor, C. S. (2012). *"Interplay of oxytocin, vasopressin, and sex hormones in the regulation of social recognition."*. Behavioral neuroscience.

Gaesser, G. A. (2021). *"Perspective: does glycemic index matter for weight loss and obesity prevention? Examination of the evidence on "fast" compared with "slow" carbs."*. Advances in Nutrition.

Gallagher, J. C. (2023). *"Vitamin D: 100 years of discoveries, yet controversy continues."*. The Lancet Diabetes & Endocrinology.

Gallagher, M. D.-S. (2019). *Prophylactic antibiotics to prevent surgical site infection after breast cancer surgery*. Cochrane Database of Systematic Reviews.

Gallo, A. e. (2023). *"Lactose malabsorption and intolerance: What is the correct management in older adults?."*. Clinical Nutrition.

Gallucci, G. e. (2020). *"Cardiovascular risk of smoking and benefits of smoking cessation."*. Journal of thoracic disease.

Galluzzi, L. e. (2015). *"Autophagy in malignant transformation and cancer progression."*. The EMBO journal.

Gandhi, A. e. (2020). *"Effect of a pedometer-based exercise program on cancer related fatigue and quality of life amongst patients with breast cancer receiving chemotherapy."*. Asian Pacific journal of cancer prevention.

Gannon, R. H. (2008). *"Estimates of daily net endogenous acid production in the elderly UK population: analysis of the National Diet and Nutrition Survey (NDNS) of British adults aged 65 years and over."*. British journal of nutrition.

Gao, Q. e. (2022). *"Prevalence and prognostic value of sarcopenic obesity in patients with cancer: a systematic review and meta-analysis."*. Nutrition.

García-Fernández, G. e. (2023). *"Effectiveness of including weight management in smoking cessation treatments: a meta-analysis of behavioral interventions."*. Addictive Behaviors.

Garland, M. e. (2018). *The impact of obesity on outcomes for patients undergoing mastectomy using the ACS-NSQIP data set.* Breast Cancer Research and Treatment.

Garrett, K. e. (2011). "*Differences in sleep disturbance and fatigue between patients with breast and prostate cancer at the initiation of radiation therapy.*". Journal of pain and symptom management.

Garvey, M. (2023). "*The association between dysbiosis and neurological conditions often manifesting with chronic pain.*". Biomedicines.

Gathani, T. e. (2017). "*Lifelong vegetarianism and breast cancer risk: a large multicentre case control study in India.*". BMC Women's Health.

Gavilan, E. e. (2023). "*Efficacy of Presurgical Interventions to Promote Smoking Cessation: A Systematic Review.*". Anesthesia & Analgesia.

Ge, X. e. (2017). "*Antibiotics-induced depletion of mice microbiota induces changes in host serotonin biosynthesis and intestinal motility.*". Journal of translational medicine.

Ge, X. e. (2022). *Predicting hyperglycemia among patients receiving alpelisib plus fulvestrant for metastatic breast cancer.* Journal of Clinical Oncology .

Gehring, J. e. (2021). "*Consumption of ultra-processed foods by pesco-vegetarians, vegetarians, and vegans: associations with duration and age at diet initiation.*". The Journal of nutrition.

Geiker, N. R. (2020). "*Impact of whole dairy matrix on musculoskeletal health and aging–current knowledge and research gaps.*". Osteoporosis International.

Genkinger, J. M. (2013). "*Consumption of dairy and meat in relation to breast cancer risk in the Black Women's Health Study.*". Cancer Causes & Control .

Gentilucci, M. M. (2020). "*Effects of Prophylactic Lipofilling After Radiotherapy Compared to Non–Fat Injected Breasts: A Randomized, Objective Study.*". Aesthetic surgery journal.

Georgescu, T. D. (2021). "*Role of serotonin in body weight, insulin secretion and glycaemic control.*". Journal of Neuroendocrinology.

Gera, R. e. (2018). *Does the use of hair dyes increase the risk of developing breast cancer? A meta-analysis and review of the literature.* Anticancer research.

Gera, T. H. (2012). *"Effect of iron-fortified foods on hematologic and biological outcomes: systematic review of randomized controlled trials."*. The American journal of clinical nutrition.

Gerald, L. (2018). *Human Biochemistry: Catabolism of Amino Acids.* Elsevier.

Gevorgyan, A. e. (2016). *"Body mass index and clinical benefit of fulvestrant in postmenopausal women with advanced breast cancer."*. Tumori Journal.

Gezer, C. a. (2013). *"Orthorexia nervosa: is it a risk for female students studying nutrition and dietetics?."*. Süleyman Demirel Üniversitesi Sağlık Bilimleri Dergisi .

Giampieri, F. e. (2022). *"Organic vs conventional plant-based foods: A review."*. Food Chemistry.

Gilsing, A. M. (2011). *"Consumption of dietary fat and meat and risk of ovarian cancer in the Netherlands Cohort Study."*. The American journal of clinical nutrition.

Glavaš, M. e. (2022). *"Vasopressin and its analogues: from natural hormones to multitasking peptides."*. International journal of molecular sciences.

Godinho-Mota, J. C. (2021). *"Chemotherapy negatively impacts body composition, physical function and metabolic profile in patients with breast cancer."*. Clinical nutrition.

Godinho-Mota, J. C. (2021). *Chemotherapy negatively impacts body composition, physical function and metabolic profile in patients with breast cancer.* Clinical nutrition.

Godos, J. e. (2017). *"Vegetarianism and breast, colorectal and prostate cancer risk: an overview and meta-analysis of cohort studies."*. Journal of Human Nutrition and Dietetics.

Goel, S. A. (2018). *"Effect of alcohol consumption on cardiovascular health."*. Current cardiology reports.

Goeptar, A. R. (1997). *"Impact of digestion on the antimutagenic activity of the milk protein casein."*. Nutrition Research.

Gohagan, J. K. (2000). *"The prostate, lung, colorectal and ovarian (PLCO) cancer screening trial of the National Cancer Institute: history, organization, and status."*. Controlled clinical trials.

Goldberg, C. e. (2024). *"Ovarian Suppression: Early Menopause, Late Effects."*. Current Oncology Reports.

Goldsmith, C. e. (2011). *"Large breast size as a risk factor for late adverse effects of breast radiotherapy: is residual dose inhomogeneity, despite 3D treatment planning and delivery, the main explanation?"*. Radiotherapy and Oncology.

Gollhofer, S. M. (2015). *"Factors influencing participation in a randomized controlled resistance exercise intervention study in breast cancer patients during radiotherapy."*. BMC cancer.

González Delgado, S. e. (2022). *"Interplay between serotonin, immune response, and intestinal dysbiosis in inflammatory bowel disease."*. International Journal of Molecular Sciences.

Gonzalez, J. T. (2024). *"Are all sugars equal? Role of the food source in physiological responses to sugars with an emphasis on fruit and fruit juice."*. European Journal of Nutrition.

Gorber, S. C. (2007). *"A comparison of direct vs. self-report measures for assessing height, weight and body mass index: a systematic review."*. Obesity reviews.

Gorissen, S. H. (2015). *"The muscle protein synthetic response to food ingestion."*. Meat science.

Gosse, M. A. (2014). *"How accurate is self-reported BMI?"*. Nutrition bulletin.

Gou, Y.-J. e. (2013). *"Alcohol consumption and breast Cancer survival: a Metaanalysis of cohort studies."*. Asian Pacific Journal of Cancer Prevention.

Gouin, J.-P. e. (2012). *"Plasma vasopressin and interpersonal functioning."*. Biological psychology.

Gouws, C. a. (2020). *"What are the dangers of drug interactions with herbal medicines?"*. Expert opinion on drug metabolism & toxicology.

Grasmann, G. e. (2019). *Gluconeogenesis in cancer cells–repurposing of a starvation-induced metabolic pathway?* Biochimica et Biophysica Acta - Reviews on Cancer.

Greenlee, H. e. (2017). *BMI, lifestyle factors and taxane-induced neuropathy in breast cancer patients: the pathways study."* . Journal of the National Cancer Institute.

Gregory, S. e. (2023). *"Mediterranean diet and structural neuroimaging biomarkers of Alzheimer's and cerebrovascular disease: A systematic review."*. Experimental gerontology.

Grimm, S. e. (2014). *"Early life stress modulates oxytocin effects on limbic system during acute psychosocial stress."*. Social cognitive and affective neuroscience.

Griswold, M. G. (2018). *"Alcohol use and burden for 195 countries and territories, 1990–2016: a systematic analysis for the Global Burden of Disease Study 2016."*. The Lancet.

Gruber, A. G. (2023). *"Adherence to the Enhanced Recovery After Surgery (ERAS) protocol in breast reconstruction plastic surgery."*. Revista Brasileira de Cirurgia Plástica.

Grządka, E. e. (2024). *"Do You Know What You Drink? Comparative Research on the Contents of Radioisotopes and Heavy Metals in Different Types of Tea from Various Parts of the World."*. Foods.

Guenancia, C. e. (2016). *Obesity as a risk factor for anthracyclines and trastuzumab cardiotoxicity in breast cancer: a systematic review and meta-analysis.* Journal of Clinical Oncology.

Guo, S. e. (2023). *"Effects of exercise on chemotherapy-induced peripheral neuropathy in cancer patients: a systematic review and meta-analysis."*. Journal of Cancer Survivorship.

Gupta, R. e. (2018). *"A systematic review on association between smokeless tobacco & cardiovascular diseases."*. Indian Journal of Medical Research.

Gutiérrez Hermoso, L. e. (2020). *"The importance of alexithymia in post-surgery. Differences on body image and psychological adjustment in breast cancer patients."*. Frontiers in psychology.

Gwin, J. A. (2020). *"Muscle protein synthesis and whole-body protein turnover responses to ingesting essential amino acids, intact protein, and protein-containing mixed meals with considerations for energy deficit."*. Nutrients.

Hägele, F. A. (2019). *"Appetite control is improved by acute increases in energy turnover at different levels of energy balance."*. The Journal of Clinical Endocrinology & Metabolism.

Händel, M. N. (2020). *"Processed meat intake and incidence of colorectal cancer: a systematic review and meta-analysis of prospective observational studies."*. European Journal of Clinical Nutrition.

Hall, L. H. (2022). *"Strategies to self-manage side-effects of adjuvant endocrine therapy among breast cancer survivors: an umbrella review of empirical evidence and clinical guidelines."*. Journal of Cancer Survivorship.

Hammarström, A. e. (2024). *"How do labour market conditions explain the development of mental health over the life-course? a conceptual integration of the ecological model with life-course epidemiology in an integrative review of results from the Northern Swedish Cohort."*. BMC Public Health.

Han, L. e. (2019). *"Smoking and influenza-associated morbidity and mortality: a systematic review and meta-analysis."*. Epidemiology.

Han, M. A. (2019). *"Reduction of red and processed meat intake and cancer mortality and incidence: a systematic review and meta-analysis of cohort studies."*. Annals of Internal Medicine.

Han, Z. X. (2024). *"Sleep deprivation: A risk factor for the pathogenesis and progression of Alzheimer's disease."*. Heliyon.

Hannah, J. e. (2018). *"Phosphorus in food: limitations of food composition data."*. Journal of Kidney Care.

Hanwright, P. J. (2013). *The differential effect of BMI on prosthetic versus autogenous breast reconstruction: a multivariate analysis of 12,986 patients.* The Breast.

Harborg, S. e. (2021). *Overweight and prognosis in triple-negative breast cancer patients: a systematic review and meta-analysis.* NPJ breast cancer.

Hargreaves, D. F. (1999). *"Two-week dietary soy supplementation has an estrogenic effect on normal premenopausal breast."*. The Journal of Clinical Endocrinology & Metabolism.

Harper, P. a.-F. (2006). *"Assessing anaemia and fatigue: putting theory into practice."* . Current Medical Research and Opinion.

Hasenoehrl, T. e. (2020). *"Resistance exercise and breast cancer–related lymphedema—a systematic review update and meta-analysis."*. Supportive Care in Cancer.

Hassan, H. e. (2023). *"Long-term outcomes of hysterectomy with bilateral salpingo-oophorectomy: a systematic review and meta-analysis."*. American Journal of Obstetrics and Gynecology.

Heasman, K. Z. (1985). *Weight gain during adjuvant chemotherapy for breast cancer.* Breast cancer research and treatment.

Hébuterne, X. e. (2014). *"Prevalence of malnutrition and current use of nutrition support in patients with cancer."*. Journal of Parenteral and Enteral Nutrition.

Heil, D. P. (2010). *"Acid-base balance and hydration status following consumption of mineral-based alkaline bottled water."*. Journal of the International Society of Sports Nutrition.

Hepsomali, P. e. (2020). *"Effects of oral gamma-aminobutyric acid (GABA) administration on stress and sleep in humans: A systematic review."*. Frontiers in neuroscience.

Heriseanu, A. I. (2017). *"Grazing in adults with obesity and eating disorders: A systematic review of associated clinical features and meta-analysis of prevalence."*. Clinical psychology review.

Hernandez Ruiz, A. e. (2015). *"Description of indexes based on the adherence to the Mediterranean dietary pattern: a review."*. Sociedad Española de Nutrición Parenteral y Enteral (SENPE).

Heymsfield, S. B. (2022). *"Phenotypic differences between people varying in muscularity."*. Journal of Cachexia, Sarcopenia and Muscle.

Hillam, J. S. (2017). *"Smoking as a risk factor for breast reduction: An analysis of 13,503 cases."*. Journal of Plastic, Reconstructive & Aesthetic Surgery.

Hirko, K. A. (2016). *Alcohol consumption and risk of breast cancer by molecular subtype: Prospective analysis of the nurses' health study after 26 years of follow-up."*. International journal of cancer.

Hirko, K. A. (2024). *"Lifetime alcohol consumption patterns and young-onset breast cancer by subtype among Non-Hispanic Black and White women in the Young Women's Health History Study."*. Cancer Causes & Control.

Ho, K.-S. e. (2012). *"Stopping or reducing dietary fiber intake reduces constipation and its associated symptoms."*. World Journal of Gastroenterology.

Ho, P. J. (2020). *"Impact of deviation from guideline recommended treatment on breast cancer survival in Asia."*. Scientific Reports.

Holahan, C. J. (2012). *"Wine consumption and 20-year mortality among late-life moderate drinkers."*. Journal of Studies on Alcohol and Drugs.

Hooper, L. e. (2010). *"Effects of isoflavones on breast density in pre-and post-menopausal women: a systematic review and meta-analysis of randomized controlled trials."*. Human reproduction update.

Houghton, S. C. (2021). *"Central adiposity and subsequent risk of breast cancer by menopause status."*. Journal of the National Cancer Institute.

Houghton, S. C. (2021). *"Central adiposity and subsequent risk of breast cancer by menopause status."*. JNCI: Journal of the National Cancer Institute.

Hsiao, Y.-H. e. (2015). *"Sleep disorders and increased risk of autoimmune diseases in individuals without sleep apnea."*. Sleep.

Hu, T. Z. (2018). *"Pharmacological effects and regulatory mechanisms of tobacco smoking effects on food intake and weight control."*. Journal of Neuroimmune Pharmacology.

Hu, X. e. (2019). *"Comparison of 4th ESO–ESMO international consensus guidelines for advance breast cancer and Chinese anti-cancer association committee of Breast Cancer Society guideline."*. The Breast.

Hudson, A. e. (2018). *"A review of the toxicity of compounds found in herbal dietary supplements."*. Planta medica.

Huedo-Medina, T. B. (2016). *"Methodologic quality of meta-analyses and systematic reviews on the Mediterranean diet and cardiovascular disease outcomes: a review."*. The American journal of clinical nutrition.

Huh, J. e. (2020). *"Prognostic value of skeletal muscle depletion measured on computed tomography for overall survival in patients with non-metastatic breast cancer."*. Journal of Breast Cancer.

Huo, J. e. (2016). *Post-mastectomy breast reconstruction and its subsequent complications: a comparison between obese and non-obese women with breast cancer.* Breast cancer research and treatment.

IARC. (1988). *IARC monographs on the evaluation of carcinogenic risks to humans. Volume 44. Alcohol drinking. Summary of data reported and evaluation. Lyon, France: IARC.* WHO.

Iguacel, I. e. (2019). *"Veganism, vegetarianism, bone mineral density, and fracture risk: a systematic review and meta-analysis.".* Nutrition reviews.

Imamura, F. e. (2018). *"Fatty acid biomarkers of dairy fat consumption and incidence of type 2 diabetes: a pooled analysis of prospective cohort studies.".* PLoS medicine.

Inglis, J. E. (2020). *Longitudinal assessment of the impact of higher body mass index on cancer-related fatigue in patients with breast cancer receiving chemotherapy.* Supportive Care in Cancer.

Ingram, I. e. (2020). *"Loneliness among people with substance use problems: A narrative systematic review.".* Drug and Alcohol Review.

Ioannides, S. J. (2014). *Effect of obesity on aromatase inhibitor efficacy in postmenopausal, hormone receptor-positive breast cancer: a systematic review.* Breast cancer research and treatment.

Ioannis, P. S. (2015). *"Graviola: A systematic review on its anticancer properties.".* Am J Cancer Prev.

Ismail, A. e. (2019). *"Aflatoxins in plant-based foods.".* Plant and Human Health, Volume 2: Phytochemistry and Molecular Aspects.

Itumalla, R. e. (2024). *"Smokeless tobacco consumption among women of reproductive age: a systematic review and meta-analysis.".* BMC Public Health.

Iwase, T. e. (2016). *"Impact of body fat distribution on neoadjuvant chemotherapy outcomes in advanced breast cancer patients.".* Cancer medicine.

Iwase, T. e. (2020). *"Quality and quantity of visceral fat tissue are associated with insulin resistance and survival outcomes after chemotherapy in patients with breast cancer.".* Breast cancer research and treatment.

Iwase, T. e. (2021). *Body composition and breast cancer risk and treatment: mechanisms and impact.* Breast cancer research and treatment.

Iyengar, N. M. (2019). *"Association of body fat and risk of breast cancer in postmenopausal women with normal body mass index: a secondary analysis of a randomized clinical trial and observational study.".* JAMA oncology.

Iyengar, N. M. (2019). *Association of body fat and risk of breast cancer in postmenopausal women with normal body mass index: a secondary analysis of a randomized clinical trial and observational study.* JAMA oncology.

Izzi, B. e. (2020). *"Beyond haemostasis and thrombosis: platelets in depression and its co-morbidities.".* International Journal of Molecular Sciences.

Jørgensen, H. e. (2003). *"Serotonin receptors involved in vasopressin and oxytocin secretion.".* Journal of neuroendocrinology.

Jahrami, H. A. (2020). *"A systematic review, meta-analysis, and meta-regression of the impact of diurnal intermittent fasting during Ramadan on body weight in healthy subjects aged 16 years and above.".* European journal of nutrition.

Jain, N. S. (2023). *"Sarcopenia Best Predicts Complications in Free Flap Breast Reconstruction.".* Plastic and Reconstructive Surgery–Global Open.

Jain, P. e. (2020). *"Weight gain after smoking cessation and lifestyle strategies to reduce it.".* Epidemiology.

Jaiswal, A. K. (2020). *"Nutritional significance of processed potato products.".* Potato: Nutrition and Food Security.

Jang, M. K. (2022). *"Body composition change during neoadjuvant chemotherapy for breast cancer.".* Frontiers in Oncology.

Jang, M. K. (2022). *"Does neoadjuvant chemotherapy regimen affect sarcopenia status in patients with breast cancer?".* The Breast .

Jang, M. K. (2023). *"Hematologic toxicities, sarcopenia, and body composition change in breast cancer patients undergoing neoadjuvant chemotherapy.".* Supportive Care in Cancer.

Jang, M. K. (2023). *"The effectiveness of Sarcopenia interventions for cancer patients receiving chemotherapy: A systematic review and meta-analysis.".* Cancer Nursing.

Jang, M. K. (2023). *"The effectiveness of Sarcopenia interventions for cancer patients receiving chemotherapy: A systematic review and meta-analysis."*. Cancer nursing.

Janssen, H. e. (2023). *"Cold indoor temperatures and their association with health and well-being: a systematic literature review."*. Public health.

Jarvis, H. e. (2022). *"Does moderate alcohol consumption accelerate the progression of liver disease in NAFLD? A systematic review and narrative synthesis."*.

Javed, A. A. (2022). *"Age-appropriate BMI cut-points for cardiometabolic health risk: a cross-sectional analysis of the Canadian Longitudinal Study on Aging."*. International journal of obesity.

Jayasinghe, M. e. (2024). *"The Role of Diet in the Management of Irritable Bowel Syndrome: A Comprehensive Review."*. Cureus.

Jayes, L. e. (2016). *"SmokeHaz: systematic reviews and meta-analyses of the effects of smoking on respiratory health."*. Chest.

Jelaković, B. e. (2023). *"Worldwide trends in underweight and obesity from 1990 to 2022: a pooled analysis of 3663 population-representative studies with 222 million children, adolescents, and adults."*. The Lancet.

Jeon, Y. W. (2021). *"Intermuscular fat density as a novel prognostic factor in breast cancer patients treated with adjuvant chemotherapy."*. Breast Cancer Research and Treatment.

Jermini, M. e. (2019). *"Complementary medicine use during cancer treatment and potential herb-drug interactions from a cross-sectional study in an academic centre."*. Scientific reports.

Jiang, C. Q. (2020). *"Smoking increases the risk of infectious diseases: A narrative review."*. Tobacco Induced Diseases.

Jiang, W. e. (2023). *"The global, regional and National Burden of pancreatic Cancer attributable to smoking, 1990 to 2019: a systematic analysis from the global burden of disease study 2019."*. International Journal of Environmental Research and Public Health.

Jogerst, K. e. (2023). *"How to teach ERAS protocols: surgical residents' perspectives and perioperative practices for breast surgery patients."*.

Global Surgical Education-Journal of the Association for Surgical Education.

Jones, M. E. (2019). *Night shift work and risk of breast cancer in women: the Generations Study cohort.* British journal of cancer.

Jonnakuty, C. a. (2008). "What do we know about serotonin?.". Journal of cellular physiology.

Joshi, A. e. (2022). "Role of the striatal dopamine, GABA and opioid systems in mediating feeding and fat intake.". Neuroscience & Biobehavioral Reviews.

Ju, Y. H. (2006). "Genistein stimulates growth of human breast cancer cells in a novel, postmenopausal animal model, with low plasma estradiol concentrations." . Carcinogenesis.

Ju, Y. H. (2008). "Dietary genistein negates the inhibitory effect of letrozole on the growth of aromatase-expressing estrogen-dependent human breast cancer cells (MCF-7Ca) in vivo.". Carcinogenesis.

Jubber, I. e. (2023). "Epidemiology of bladder cancer in 2023: a systematic review of risk factors.". European urology.

Jung, A. Y. (2021). *Postdiagnosis weight change is associated with poorer survival in breast cancer survivors: a prospective population‐based patient cohort study.* International journal of cancer.

Jung, D. e. (2016). "Longitudinal association of poor sleep quality with chemotherapy-induced nausea and vomiting in patients with breast cancer.". Psychosomatic medicine.

Kahneman, D. O. (2021). *Noise: A flaw in human judgment.* Hachette UK.

Kale, Y. S. (2019). "Effect of using tobacco on taste perception.". Journal of family medicine and primary care.

Kalinowski, A. a. (2016). "Governmental standard drink definitions and low‐risk alcohol consumption guidelines in 37 countries.". Addiction.

Kalinyak, J. E. (2014). *Breast cancer detection using high-resolution breast PET compared to whole-body PET or PET/CT.* European journal of nuclear medicine and molecular imaging.

Kamińska, M. S. (2023). *"The impact of whey protein supplementation on sarcopenia progression among the elderly: a systematic review and meta-analysis."*. Nutrients.

Kancherla, B. S. (2020). *"Sleep, fatigue and burnout among physicians: an American Academy of Sleep Medicine position statement."*. Journal of Clinical Sleep Medicine.

Kancherla, B. S. (2020). *"Sleep, fatigue and burnout among physicians: an American Academy of Sleep Medicine position statement."*.

Karatas, F. e. (2017). *Obesity is an independent prognostic factor of decreased pathological complete response to neoadjuvant chemotherapy in breast cancer patients.* The Breast.

Kareklas, K. a. (2024). *Oxytocin and Social Isolation: Nonapeptide Regulation of Social Homeostasis."*. Neuroendocrinology of Behavior and Emotions: Environmental and Social Factors Affecting Behavior. Cham: Springer International Publishing.

Karpman, S. (1968). *"Fairy tales and script drama analysis."*. Transactional analysis bulletin.

Katidi, A. e. (2023). *"Nutritional quality of plant-based meat and dairy imitation products and comparison with animal-based counterparts."*. Nutrients.

Kayser, K. C. (2022). *"Predicting and mitigating fatigue effects due to sleep deprivation: A review."*. Frontiers in Neuroscience.

Keeton, J. T. (2017). *"'Red'and 'white'meats—terms that lead to confusion."*. Animal Frontiers.

Keilani, M. e. (2016). *"Resistance exercise and secondary lymphedema in breast cancer survivors—a systematic review."*. Supportive Care in Cancer.

Keith, S. W. (2011). *"Use of self-reported height and weight biases the body mass index–mortality association."*. International journal of obesity.

Kennedy, C. D. (2019). *"The cardiovascular effects of electronic cigarettes: a systematic review of experimental studies."*. Preventive medicine.

Keramaris, A. E. (2022). *"Pontic Greek cuisine: the most common foods, ingredients, and dishes presented in cookbooks and folklore literature."*. Journal of Ethnic Foods.

Kerner, J. a. (2000). *"Fatty acid import into mitochondria."*. Biochimica et Biophysica Acta (BBA)-molecular and cell biology of Lipids.

Kershbaum, A. e. (1963). *"The role of catecholamines in the free fatty acid response to cigarette smoking."*. Circulation.

Keys, A. (1980). *Seven countries: a multivariate analysis of death and coronary heart disease.* Harvard University Press.

Keys, A. e. (1950). *"The biology of human starvation.(2 vols)."*.

Keys, A. e. (1950). *"The biology of human starvation, Vols. 1 & 2."*.

Keys, A. e. (1963). *"Coronary heart disease among Minnesota business and professional men followed fifteen years."*. Circulation.

Kharbanda, C. S. (2022). *"Role and significance of ghrelin and leptin in hunger, satiety, and energy homeostasis.* Journal of the Scientific Society.

Khoramdad, M. e. (2020). *"Association between passive smoking and cardiovascular disease: A systematic review and meta-analysis."*. IUBMB life.

Khosrow-Khavar, F. (2020). *Cardiovascular Safety of Aromatase Inhibitors in Post-Menopausal Women with Breast Cancer.* McGill University (Canada).

Kim, H. J. (2024). *"Smoking cessation and risk of metabolic syndrome: A meta-analysis."*. Medicine.

Kim, J. Y. (2009). *"Garlic intake and cancer risk: an analysis using the Food and Drug Administration's evidence-based review system for the scientific evaluation of health claims."*. The American journal of clinical nutrition.

Kim, S. e. (2022). *"Association of preoperative sarcopenia with adverse outcomes of breast reconstruction using deep inferior epigastric artery perforator flap."*. Annals of Surgical Oncology.

Kimble, R. e. (2023). *"Effects of a mediterranean diet on the gut microbiota and microbial metabolites: A systematic review of randomized controlled trials and observational studies."*. Critical Reviews in Food Science and Nutrition.

King, E. a. (2023). *"Associations between level of interest in nutrition, knowledge of nutrition, and prevalence of orthorexia traits among undergraduate students."*. Nutrition and Health.

Kipnis, V. e. (2002). *"Bias in dietary-report instruments and its implications for nutritional epidemiology."*. Public health nutrition.

Kirkham, A. A. (2019). *"Curing breast cancer and killing the heart: a novel model to explain elevated cardiovascular disease and mortality risk among women with early stage breast cancer."*. Progress in Cardiovascular Diseases.

Klasson, S. e. (2016). *"Smoking increases donor site complications in breast reconstruction with DIEP flap."*. Journal of plastic surgery and hand surgery.

Klek, S. e. (2014). *Perioperative immunonutrition in surgical cancer patients: a summary of a decade of research.* World journal of surgery.

Klement, R. J. (2020). *"Ketogenic diets in medical oncology: a systematic review with focus on clinical outcomes."*. Medical Oncology.

Knight, J. A. (2017). *"Alcohol consumption and cigarette smoking in combination: A predictor of contralateral breast cancer risk in the WECARE study."*. International journal of cancer.

Knowles, O. E. (2024). *"The interactive effect of sustained sleep restriction and resistance exercise on skeletal muscle transcriptomics in young females."*. Physiological Genomics.

Knowlton, S. E. (2024). *"Medical and Cardiac Risk Stratification and Exercise Prescription in Persons With Cancer."*. American Journal of Physical Medicine & Rehabilitation.

Knuppel, A. e. (2020). *"Meat intake and cancer risk: prospective analyses in UK Biobank."*. International Journal of Epidemiology.

Ko, D. T. (2016). *"High-density lipoprotein cholesterol and cause-specific mortality in individuals without previous cardiovascular conditions: the CANHEART study."*. Journal of the American College of Cardiology.

Ko, H. e. (2021). *"Low-level alcohol consumption and cancer mortality."*. Scientific reports.

Koeder, C. a.-C. (2024). *"Vegan nutrition: a preliminary guide for health professionals."*. Critical reviews in food science and nutrition.

Kogawa, T. e. (2018). *"Impact of change in body mass index during neoadjuvant chemotherapy and survival among breast cancer subtypes."*. Breast cancer research and treatment.

Kojima, M. a. (2002). *"Ghrelin, an orexigenic signaling molecule from the gastrointestinal tract."*. Current opinion in pharmacology.

Kolahdooz, F. e. (2010). *"Meat, fish, and ovarian cancer risk: results from 2 Australian case-control studies, a systematic review, and meta-analysis."* . The American journal of clinical nutrition.

Koopman, R. (2007). *"Role of amino acids and peptides in the molecular signaling in skeletal muscle after resistance exercise."*. International journal of sport nutrition and exercise metabolism.

Koopman, R. e. (2005). *"A single session of resistance exercise enhances insulin sensitivity for at least 24 h in healthy men."*. European journal of applied physiology.

Korde, L. A. (2009). *"Childhood soy intake and breast cancer risk in Asian American women."*. Cancer Epidemiology Biomarkers & Prevention.

Kornitzer, M. e. (1981). *"The Belgian Heart Disease Prevention Project: Type "A" behavior pattern and the prevalence of coronary heart disease."*. Psychosomatic Medicine.

Kotfis, K. e. (2020). *"The effect of preoperative carbohydrate loading on clinical and biochemical outcomes after cardiac surgery: A systematic review and meta-analysis of randomized trials."*. Nutrients.

Koundouros, N. a. (2020). *"Reprogramming of fatty acid metabolism in cancer."*. British journal of cancer .

Kovář, J. a. (2015). *"Moderate alcohol consumption and triglyceridemia."*. Physiological research.

Kowalczyk, L. e. (2021). *"Radiotherapy-induced fatigue in breast cancer patients."*. Breast Care.

Krasniqi, E. e. (2020). *"Impact of BMI on HER2+ metastatic breast cancer patients treated with pertuzumab and/or trastuzumab emtansine. Real-world evidence."*. Journal of Cellular Physiology.

Krebs, H. (1960). *"Biochemical aspects of ketosis."*.
Krebs, P. e. (2018). *"Stages of change and psychotherapy outcomes: A review and meta-analysis."*. Journal of clinical psychology.
Krebs, P. e. (2018). *"Stages of change and psychotherapy outcomes: A review and meta-analysis."*. Journal of clinical psychology.
Kristensen, L. a. (2001). *"The effect of processing temperature and addition of mono-and di-valent salts on the heme-nonheme-iron ratio in meat."*. Food chemistry.
Krnic, M. e. (2011). *"Comparison of acute effects of red wine, beer and vodka against hyperoxia-induced oxidative stress and increase in arterial stiffness in healthy humans."*. Atherosclerosis.
Kroemer, G. a.-L. (2014). *Entosis, a key player in cancer cell competition.* Cell Research.
Kromhout, D. e. (1989). *"Food consumption patterns in the 1960s in seven countries."*. The American journal of clinical nutrition.
Kruger, C. a. (2018). *"Red meat and colon cancer: a review of mechanistic evidence for heme in the context of risk assessment methodology."*. Food and Chemical Toxicology.
Kuśnierczyk, P. (2023). *"Genetic differences between smokers and never-smokers with lung cancer."*. Frontiers in Immunology.
Kudiarasu, C. e. (2023). *"What are the most effective exercise, physical activity and dietary interventions to improve body composition in women diagnosed with or at high-risk of breast cancer? A systematic review and network meta-analysis."*. Cancer.
Kujath, A. S. (2015). *"Oxytocin levels are lower in premenopausal women with type 1 diabetes mellitus compared with matched controls."*. Diabetes/metabolism research and reviews.
Kumar, N. e. (2024). *"The unique risk factor profile of triple negative breast cancer: a comprehensive meta-analysis."*. Journal of the National Cancer Institute.
Kumar, V. e. (2009). *"Human muscle protein synthesis and breakdown during and after exercise."*. Journal of applied physiology.
Kuratko, C. e. (2016). *"Systematic Reviews of Current Literature Fail to Establish Dietary Benzo [a] pyrene, Heterocyclic Aromatic Amines, or Heme Iron as Mechanisms Linking Red and

Processed Meat Consumption with Cancer Risk.". The FASEB Journal.

Kuroi, K. e. (2006). *"Evidence-based risk factors for seroma formation in breast surgery."*. Japanese journal of clinical oncology.

Kwan, M. L. (2010). *"Alcohol consumption and breast cancer recurrence and survival among women with early-stage breast cancer: the life after cancer epidemiology study."*. Journal of clinical Oncology.

Lac, A. a. (2022). *"Development and validation of the Drama Triangle Scale: are you a victim, rescuer, or persecutor?."*. Journal of interpersonal violence.

Lahart, I. M. (2015). *"Physical activity, risk of death and recurrence in breast cancer survivors: a systematic review and meta-analysis of epidemiological studies."*. Acta oncologica.

Lambertini, M. e. (2018). *"The BCY3/BCC 2017 survey on physicians' knowledge, attitudes and practice towards fertility and pregnancy-related issues in young breast cancer patients."*. The Breast.

Lamon, S. e. (2021). *"The effect of acute sleep deprivation on skeletal muscle protein synthesis and the hormonal environment."*. Physiological reports.

Lancaster, T. a. (2017). *"Individual behavioural counselling for smoking cessation."*. Cochrane database of systematic reviews.

Lane, J. e. (2021). *"Ketogenic diet for cancer: critical assessment and research recommendations."*. Nutrients.

Lange, M. G. (2024). *"Metabolic changes with intermittent fasting."*. Journal of Human Nutrition and Dietetics.

Lassale, C. e. (2019). *"Healthy dietary indices and risk of depressive outcomes: a systematic review and meta-analysis of observational studies."*. Molecular psychiatry.

Lau, K. e. (2017). *"Bridging the gap between gut microbial dysbiosis and cardiovascular diseases."*. Nutrients.

Lau, W. K.-W. (2023). *"The differential effect of oxytocin on mindfulness in people with different resilience level."*. Mindfulness.

Lavery, J. A. (2024). *"Association of exercise with pan-cancer incidence and overall survival."*. Cancer Cell.

Lavoie, B. J. (2017). *"Regulation of bone metabolism by serotonin."*. Understanding the Gut-Bone Signaling Axis: Mechanisms and Therapeutic Implications.

Lawson, E. A. (2011). *"Appetite-regulating hormones cortisol and peptide YY are associated with disordered eating psychopathology, independent of body mass index."*. European journal of endocrinology.

le Riche, W. H. (1981). *"Foods, fads and fallacies."*. Modern Medicine.

LeBlanc, V. R. (2015). *"Predictable chaos: a review of the effects of emotions on attention, memory and decision making."*. Advances in Health Sciences Education.

Lee, A. C. (2022). *"Impact of obesity on safety outcomes and treatment modifications with ado-trastuzumab emtansine in breast cancer patients."*. Journal of Oncology Pharmacy Practice.

Lee, A. N. (2004). *"Activation of autoimmunity following use of immunostimulatory herbal supplements."*. Archives of Dermatology.

Lee, B. S.-W.-K. (2015). *"Efficacy of vitamin C supplements in prevention of cancer: a meta-analysis of randomized controlled trials."*. Korean Journal of Family Medicine.

Lee, J. a.-G. (2020). *"Effects of exercise interventions on breast cancer patients during adjuvant therapy: a systematic review and meta-analysis of randomized controlled trials."*. Cancer nursing.

Lee, J. e. (2021). *"Sedentary work and breast cancer risk: A systematic review and meta-analysis."*. Journal of occupational health.

Lee, M. H. (2018). *"Dairy food consumption is associated with a lower risk of the metabolic syndrome and its components: a systematic review and meta-analysis."*. British Journal of Nutrition.

Lee, P. N. (2012). *"Systematic review with meta-analysis of the epidemiological evidence in the 1900s relating smoking to lung cancer."*. BMC cancer.

Lee, S. e. (2018). *"Microbiological safety of processed meat products formulated with low nitrite concentration—A review."*. Asian-Australasian journal of animal sciences.

Lee-Kwan, S. H. (2017). *"Disparities in state-specific adult fruit and vegetable consumption—United States, 2015.* Morbidity and mortality weekly report.

Lemieux, J. e. (2013). *"Alcohol and HER2 polymorphisms as risk factor for cardiotoxicity in breast cancer treated with trastuzumab.".* Anticancer research.

Leng, G. e. (2008). *"Oxytocin and appetite.".* Progress in brain research.

Levy, A. G. (2018). *"Prevalence of and factors associated with patient nondisclosure of medically relevant information to clinicians.".* JAMA network open .

Levy, M. A. (2015). *"Predictors of vitamin D status in subjects that consume a vitamin D supplement.".* European journal of clinical nutrition.

Lewis, L. e. (2024). *"Body composition and chemotherapy toxicities in breast cancer: a systematic review of the literature.".* Journal of Cancer Survivorship.

Lewis-Smith, H. P. (2018). *"A pilot study of a body image intervention for breast cancer survivors.".* Body image.

Leysen, L. e. (2017). *Risk factors of pain in breast cancer survivors: a systematic review and meta-analysis.* Supportive Care in Cancer.

Leysen, L. e. (2019). *"Prevalence and risk factors of sleep disturbances in breast cancersurvivors: systematic review and meta-analyses.".* Supportive Care in Cancer.

Li et al, 2. (n.d.). *Li, Christopher I., et al.* "Alcohol consumption and risk of postmenopausal breast cancer by subtype: the women's health initiative observational study." Journal of the National Cancer Institute 102.18 (2010): 1422-1431.

Li, C. I. (2010). *"Alcohol consumption and risk of postmenopausal breast cancer by subtype: the women's health initiative observational study.".* Journal of the National Cancer Institute.

Li, T. Y. (2021). *"Comparison of human bone mineral densities in subjects on plant-based and omnivorous diets: a systematic review and meta-analysis.".* Archives of Osteoporosis.

Li, X. e. (2023). *The effect of exercise on weight and body composition of breast cancer patients undergoing chemotherapy: a systematic review.* Cancer Nursing.

Li, X. e. (2024). *"The effect of exercise on weight and body composition of breast cancer patients undergoing chemotherapy: a systematic review."*. Cancer Nursing.

Li, Y. e. (2023). *"Global prevalence of Helicobacter pylori infection between 1980 and 2022: a systematic review and meta-analysis."*. The lancet Gastroenterology & hepatology.

Li, Y. W.-D. (2021). *"Effect of physical activity on the association between dietary fiber and constipation: evidence from the national health and nutrition examination survey 2005-2010."*. Journal of neurogastroenterology and motility.

Liang, J. e. (2018). *"Biomarkers of dairy fat intake and risk of cardiovascular disease: A systematic review and meta analysis of prospective studies."*. Critical reviews in food science and nutrition.

Liang, Z. e. (2023). *"Comparative efficacy of four exercise types on obesity-related outcomes in breast cancer survivors: A Bayesian network meta-analysis."*. European Journal of Oncology Nursing.

Ligorio, F. e. (2021). *"Targeting lipid metabolism is an emerging strategy to enhance the efficacy of anti-HER2 therapies in HER2-positive breast cancer."*. Cancer Letters.

Lin, C. J. (2012). *"Accuracy and reliability of self-reported weight and height in the Sister Study."*. Public health nutrition.

Lin, J. e. (2020). *"Associations of short sleep duration with appetite-regulating hormones and adipokines: A systematic review and meta-analysis."*. Obesity Reviews.

Lindson, N. e. (2024). *"Electronic cigarettes for smoking cessation."*. Cochrane Database of Systematic Reviews.

Lipsett, A. e. (2017). *"The impact of exercise during adjuvant radiotherapy for breast cancer on fatigue and quality of life: A systematic review and meta-analysis."*. The breast.

Litton, J. K. (2008). *Relationship between obesity and pathologic response to neoadjuvant chemotherapy among women with operable breast cancer.* Journal of Clinical Oncology.

Litvin, Y. a. (2013). *"The involvement of oxytocin and vasopressin in fear and anxiety."*. Oxytocin, Vasopressin and Related Peptides in the Regulation of Behavior.

Liu, L. e. (2022). *"Metabolic efficacy of time-restricted eating in adults: a systematic review and meta-analysis of randomized controlled trials."*. The Journal of Clinical Endocrinology & Metabolism.

Liu, X. A. (2018). *"Vitamin D deficiency and insufficiency among US adults: prevalence, predictors and clinical implications."*. British Journal of Nutrition.

Liu, Y. e. (2017). *Obesity and survival in the neoadjuvant breast cancer setting: Role of tumor subtype and race.* Journal of Clinical Oncology.

Liu, Y. e. (2023). *"Effectiveness of Nonpharmacologic Interventions for Chemotherapy-Related Cognitive Impairment in Breast Cancer Patients: A Systematic Review and Network Meta-analysis."*. Cancer nursing.

Liyanage, T. e. (2016). *"Effects of the Mediterranean diet on cardiovascular outcomes—a systematic review and meta-analysis."*. PloS one.

Lizarraga, I. M. (2021). *"Surgical decision-making surrounding contralateral prophylactic mastectomy: comparison of treatment goals, preferences, and psychosocial outcomes from a multicenter survey of breast cancer patients."*. Annals of surgical oncology.

Lombardi-Boccia, G. B.-D. (2002). *"Total heme and non-heme iron in raw and cooked meats."*. Journal of Food Science.

Lotfi, K. e. (2022). *"Adherence to the Mediterranean diet, five-year weight change, and risk of overweight and obesity: a systematic review and dose–response meta-analysis of prospective cohort studies."*. Advances in Nutrition.

Lubinski, J. e. (2011). *"Selenium and the risk of cancer in BRCA1 carriers."*. Hereditary cancer in clinical practice.

Lucerón-Lucas-Torres, M. e. (2023). *"Association between wine consumption with cardiovascular disease and cardiovascular mortality: a systematic review and meta-analysis."*. Nutrients.

Lucius, K. a. (2019). *"Combining immunotherapy and natural immune stimulants: mechanisms and clinical implications."*. Journal of Cancer Research and Clinical Oncology.

Ludwig, H. e. (2015). *"Iron metabolism and iron supplementation in cancer patients."*. Wiener Klinische Wochenschrift.

Ludzki, A. C. (2022). *"One week of overeating upregulates angiogenic and lipolytic gene expression in human subcutaneous adipose tissue from exercise trained and untrained adults."*. Applied Physiology, Nutrition, and Metabolism.

Luís, C. e. (2023). *Breast Cancer Molecular Subtypes Differentially Express Gluconeogenic Rate-Limiting Enzymes—Obesity as a Crucial Player.* Cancers.

Lundahl, B. e. (2013). *"Motivational interviewing in medical care settings: a systematic review and meta-analysis of randomized controlled trials."*. Patient education and counseling.

Luo, J. e. (2014). *"Systematic review with meta-analysis: meat consumption and the risk of hepatocellular carcinoma."*. Alimentary pharmacology & therapeutics.

Lynch, S. R. (1994). *"Inhibitory effect of a soybean-protein–related moiety on iron absorption in humans."*. The American journal of clinical nutrition.

Møller, A. e. (2019). *"Attenuation of dopamine-induced GABA release in problem gamblers."*. Brain and behavior.

Müller, M. e. (2018). *"Manual lymphatic drainage and quality of life in patients with lymphoedema and mixed oedema: a systematic review of randomised controlled trials."*. Quality of life research.

Macaione, I. e. (2020). *Impact of BMI on preoperative axillary ultrasound assessment in patients with early breast cancer.* Anticancer Research.

Maestrini, S. e. (2018). *"Plasma oxytocin concentration in pre-and postmenopausal women: its relationship with obesity, body composition and metabolic variables."*. Obesity Facts.

Magidman, P. e. (1962). *"Fatty acids of cows' milk. A. Techniques employed in supplementing gas-liquid chromatography for identification of fatty acids."*. Journal of the American Oil Chemists' Society.

Mancini, J. G. (2016). *"Systematic review of the Mediterranean diet for long-term weight loss."*. The American journal of medicine.
Mancini, J. G. (2016). *"Systematic review of the Mediterranean diet for long-term weight loss."*. The American journal of medicine.
Mandrioli, D. C. (2016). *"Relationship between research outcomes and risk of bias, study sponsorship, and author financial conflicts of interest in reviews of the effects of artificially sweetened beverages on weight outcomes: a systematic review of reviews."*. PloS one.
Manouchehri, E. e. (2021). *Night-shift work duration and breast cancer risk: an updated systematic review and meta-analysis.* BMC women's health.
Manson, J. E. (2019). *"Vitamin D supplements and prevention of cancer and cardiovascular disease."*. New England Journal of Medicine.
Maric, D. e. (2024). *"Effects of resistance training on sleep quality and disorders among individuals diagnosed with cancer: A systematic review and meta-analysis of randomized controlled trials."*. Cancer Medicine.
Marinescu, S. C. (2024). *"Dietary Influence on Drug Efficacy: A Comprehensive Review of Ketogenic Diet–Pharmacotherapy Interactions."*. Nutrients.
Marques-Pinto, A. e. (2018). *"Nurses' intention to leave the organization: a mediation study of professional burnout and engagement."*. The Spanish journal of psychology.
Mart, S. a. (2015). *"Red flags on pinkwashed drinks: contradictions and dangers in marketing alcohol to prevent cancer."*. Addiction.
Martel, S. e. (2021). *"Body mass index and weight change in patients with HER2-positive early breast cancer: exploratory analysis of the ALTTO BIG 2-06 trial."*. Journal of the National Comprehensive Cancer Network.
Martin, E. M. (2016). *"E-cigarette use results in suppression of immune and inflammatory-response genes in nasal epithelial cells similar to cigarette smoke."*. American Journal of Physiology-Lung Cellular and Molecular Physiology.
Martínez-González, M. Á. (2017). *"Transferability of the Mediterranean diet to non-Mediterranean countries. What is and what is not the Mediterranean diet."* . Nutrients.

Martínez-González, M. A. (2002). *"Mediterranean diet and reduction in the risk of a first acute myocardial infarction: an operational healthy dietary score."*. European journal of nutrition.

Martinez-Lacoba, R. e. (2018). *"Mediterranean diet and health outcomes: a systematic meta-review."*. European journal of public health.

Martinez-Outschoorn, U. E. (2012). *Ketone body utilization drives tumor growth and metastasis.* Cell cycle.

Martin-McGill, K. J. (2020). *"Ketogenic diets for drug-resistant epilepsy."*. Cochrane Database of Systematic Reviews.

Marvaldi, M. e. (2021). *"Anxiety, depression, trauma-related, and sleep disorders among healthcare workers during the COVID-19 pandemic: A systematic review and meta-analysis."*. Neuroscience & Biobehavioral Reviews.

Mascia, P. e. (2020). *"Maladaptive consequences of repeated intermittent exposure to uncertainty."*. Progress in neuro-psychopharmacology and biological psychiatry.

Mather, T. L. (2023). *Rates of major complications and flap loss for abdominally based breast reconstruction in obese patients are independent of WHO class of obesity.* Journal of Plastic, Reconstructive & Aesthetic Surgery.

Mathur, M. a. (1989). *"Effect of low protein diet on low dose chronic aflatoxin B1 induced hepatic injury in rhesus monkeys."*. Journal of Toxicology: Toxin Reviews.

Matthews, C. E. (2020). *"Amount and intensity of leisure-time physical activity and lower cancer risk."*. Journal of Clinical Oncology.

Matthews, L. e. (2021). *"The use of bioelectrical impedance analysis to predict post-operative complications in adult patients having surgery for cancer: A systematic review."*. Clinical Nutrition.

Maudgal, S. W. (2018). *"Alexithymia in breast cancer patients and their sisters in Seoul."*. Journal of Global Oncology.

Mazur, S. L. (2024). *"Medical Oversight and Public Trust of Medicine: Breaches of Trust."*. The Complex Role of Patient Trust in Oncology. Cham: Springer International Publishing.

McGovern, A. e. (2022). *"Efficacy of resistance training during adjuvant chemotherapy and radiation therapy in cancer care: a systematic review and meta-analysis.".* Supportive Care in Cancer.

McGrorry, A. R. (2023). *"The effects of exercise on sleep disturbances and cancer-related fatigue for female breast cancer survivors receiving adjuvant hormone therapy: a systematic review.".* Lifestyle Medicine.

McGuire, V. e. (2006). *"No increased risk of breast cancer associated with alcohol consumption among carriers of BRCA1 and BRCA2 mutations ages< 50 years.".* Cancer Epidemiology Biomarkers & Prevention.

McMichael-Phillips, D. F. (1998). *"Effects of soy-protein supplementation on epithelial proliferation in the histologically normal human breast.".* The American journal of clinical nutrition.

McQuaid, R. J. (2016). *"Relations between plasma oxytocin and cortisol: The stress buffering role of social support.".* Neurobiology of stress.

McTiernan, A. N. (2019). *"Physical activity in cancer prevention and survival: a systematic review.".* Medicine and science in sports and exercise.

McTiernan, A. N. (2019). *"Physical activity in cancer prevention and survival: a systematic review.".* Medicine and science in sports and exercise.

Medeiros Torres, D. R. (2022). *"Impact on fatigue of different types of physical exercise during adjuvant chemotherapy and radiotherapy in breast cancer: systematic review and meta-analysis.".* Supportive care in cancer.

Meeusen, V. e. (2024). *"Occupational well-being, resilience, burnout, and job satisfaction of surgical teams.".* Handbook of Perioperative and Procedural Patient Safety. Elsevier.

Mehler, P. S. (2016). *"Electrolyte and acid-base abnormalities associated with purging behaviors.".* International Journal of Eating Disorders.

Mehta, L. S. (2018). *"Cardiovascular disease and breast cancer: where these entities intersect: a scientific statement from the American Heart Association.".* Circulation.

Meini, S. e. (2021). *"The paradox of the low prevalence of current smokers among COVID-19 patients hospitalized in nonintensive care wards: results from an Italian multicenter case–control study."*. Nicotine and Tobacco Research.

Meisel, H. a. (2003). *"Biofunctional peptides from milk proteins: mineral binding and cytomodulatory effects."*. Current pharmaceutical design.

Mendes, B. G. (2020). *"From intestinal dysbiosis to alcohol-associated liver disease."*. Clinical and molecular hepatology.

Messina, M. C. (2006). *"Estimated Asian adult soy protein and isoflavone intakes."*. Nutrition and cancer.

Messina, M. V. (2024). *"Perspective: Observational studies involving low soy intake populations have limited ability for providing insight into the health effects of soybean isoflavones."*. Advances in Nutrition.

Michos, E. D. (2021). *"Vitamin D, calcium supplements, and implications for cardiovascular health: JACC focus seminar."*. Journal of the American College of Cardiology.

Milani, F. a. (2023). *"The alterations of taste and smell in smokers."*. Tabaccologia.

Miller, K. e. (2022). *"The association between guideline adherence, age and overall survival among women with non-metastatic breast cancer: A systematic review."*. Cancer Treatment Reviews.

Miller, P. E. (2014). *"Low-calorie sweeteners and body weight and composition: a meta-analysis of randomized controlled trials and prospective cohort studies."*. The American journal of clinical nutrition.

Millwood, I. Y. (2019). *"Conventional and genetic evidence on alcohol and vascular disease aetiology: a prospective study of 500 000 men and women in China."*. The Lancet.

Mineur, Y. S. (2011). *"Nicotine decreases food intake through activation of POMC neurons."*. Science.

Mirchandaney, R. L. (2023). *"Recent advances in sleep and depression."*. Current Opinion in Psychiatry.

Miyara, M. e. (2020). *"Low rate of daily smokers in patients with symptomatic COVID-19."*. MedRxiv.

Modi, N. D. (2021). *"The obesity paradox in early and advanced HER2 positive breast cancer: pooled analysis of clinical trial data."*. Breast Cancer.

Modi, N. D. (2021). *"The obesity paradox in early and advanced HER2 positive breast cancer: pooled analysis of clinical trial data."*. NPJ Breast Cancer.

Mohamady, H. M. (2017). *"Impact of moderate intensity aerobic exercise on chemotherapy-induced anemia in elderly women with breast cancer: A randomized controlled clinical trial."*. Journal of Advanced Research.

Monaco, M. E. (2017). *"Fatty acid metabolism in breast cancer subtypes."*. Oncotarget.

Monaco, M. E. (2017). *Fatty acid metabolism in breast cancer subtypes.* Oncotarget.

Moncrieff, J. e. (2023). *"The serotonin theory of depression: a systematic umbrella review of the evidence."*. Molecular psychiatry.

Monello, L. F. (1967). *"Hunger and satiety sensations in men, women, boys, and girls."*. The American Journal of Clinical Nutrition.

Monnier, L. e. (2021). *"The obesity treatment dilemma: Why dieting is both the answer and the problem? A mechanistic overview."*. Diabetes & metabolism.

Montagna, E. e. (2021). *"Assessing predictors of tamoxifen nonadherence in patients with early breast cancer."*. Patient preference and adherence.

Montagna, G. a. (2020). *"Contralateral prophylactic mastectomy in breast cancer: what to discuss with patients."*. Expert review of anticancer therapy.

Montani, J.-P. e. (2006). *"Weight cycling during growth and beyond as a risk factor for later cardiovascular diseases: the 'repeated overshoot' theory."*. International journal of obesity.

Morris, S. E. (2021). *"Burnout in psychosocial oncology clinicians: A systematic review."*. Palliative & Supportive Care.

Mortellaro, S. e. (2024). *"Quantitative and Qualitative Radiological Assessment of Sarcopenia and Cachexia in Cancer Patients: A Systematic Review."*. Journal of Personalized Medicine.

Morze, J. e. (2021). "*An updated systematic review and meta-analysis on adherence to mediterranean diet and risk of cancer.*". European journal of nutrition.

Mostofsky, E. e. (2016). "*Alcohol and immediate risk of cardiovascular events: a systematic review and dose–response meta-analysis.*". Circulation.

Mostofsky, E. e. (2024). "*Impact of Alcohol Consumption on Breast Cancer Incidence and Mortality: The Women's Health Study.*". Journal of Women's Health.

Motlaghzadeh, Y. J. (2024). "*Hypercalcemia due to vitamin D toxicity.*". Feldman and Pike's Vitamin D.

Mott, A. e. (2019). "*Effect of vitamin K on bone mineral density and fractures in adults: an updated systematic review and meta-analysis of randomised controlled trials.*". Osteoporosis International.

Mrad, M. A. (2022). "*Predictors of complications after breast reconstruction surgery: a systematic review and meta-analysis.*". Plastic and Reconstructive Surgery–Global Open.

Mrad, M. A. (2022). *Predictors of complications after breast reconstruction surgery: a systematic review and meta-analysis.* Plastic and Reconstructive Surgery–Global Open.

Mravec, B. e. (2020). "*E-cigarettes and cancer risk.*". Cancer Prevention Research.

Mullie, P. e. (2016). "*Relation between breast cancer and high glycemic index or glycemic load: a meta-analysis of prospective cohort studies.*". Critical reviews in food science and nutrition.

Murphy, J. L. (2021). "*The provision of nutritional advice and care for cancer patients: a UK national survey of healthcare professionals.*". Supportive Care in Cancer.

Murphy, K. J. (2018). "*Implementing a Mediterranean-style diet outside the Mediterranean region.*". Current atherosclerosis reports.

Murray, M. a. (2009). "*Consumer views of hunger and fullness. A qualitative approach.*". Appetite.

Muscaritoli, M. e. (2021). "*ESPEN practical guideline: Clinical Nutrition in cancer.*". Clinical Nutrition.

Muscaritoli, M. e. (2021). *ESPEN practical guideline: Clinical Nutrition in cancer.* Clinical Nutrition.

Mutschler, N. S. (2018). *"Prognostic impact of weight change during adjuvant chemotherapy in patients with high-risk early breast cancer: results from the ADEBAR study."*. Clinical breast cancer.

Myers, K. e. (2011). *"Stopping smoking shortly before surgery and postoperative complications: a systematic review and meta-analysis."*. Archives of internal medicine.

Nachit, M. e. (2023). *"AI-based CT body composition identifies myosteatosis as key mortality predictor in asymptomatic adults."*. Radiology.

Nagasaki, K. e. (2024). *"Association of sleep quality with duty hours, mental health, and medical errors among Japanese postgraduate residents: a cross-sectional study."* . Scientific Reports.

Naimi, T. S. (2017). *"Selection biases in observational studies affect associations between 'moderate' alcohol consumption and mortality."*. Addiction.

Nakagawa, T. M. (2019). *"The effects of fruit consumption in patients with hyperuricaemia or gout."*. Rheumatology.

Nakamura, H. e. (2020). *"Impact of skeletal muscle mass on complications following expander breast reconstruction."*. Journal of Plastic, Reconstructive & Aesthetic Surgery.

Narayanan, S. e. (2023). *"Medicinal mushroom supplements in cancer: a systematic review of clinical studies."*. Current oncology reports.

Naska, A. a. (2014). *"Back to the future: the Mediterranean diet paradigm."*. Nutrition, Metabolism and Cardiovascular Diseases.

Navarro, V. J. (2014). *"Hepatotoxicity induced by herbal and dietary supplements."*. Seminars in liver disease.

Neale, R. E. (2022). *"The D-Health Trial: a randomised controlled trial of the effect of vitamin D on mortality."*. The Lancet Diabetes & Endocrinology.

Nebgen, D. R. (2023). *"Care after premenopausal risk-reducing salpingo-oophorectomy in high-risk women: Scoping review and international consensus recommendations."*. BJOG: An International Journal of Obstetrics & Gynaecology.

Nechuta, S. e. (2013). "*Postdiagnosis cruciferous vegetable consumption and breast cancer outcomes: a report from the After Breast Cancer Pooling Project.*". Cancer epidemiology, biomarkers & prevention.

Nechuta, S. J. (2012). "*Soy food intake after diagnosis of breast cancer and survival: an in-depth analysis of combined evidence from cohort studies of US and Chinese women.*". The American journal of clinical nutrition.

Nedeltcheva, A. V. (2010). "*Insufficient sleep undermines dietary efforts to reduce adiposity.*". Annals of internal medicine.

Neri, L. d. (2024). "*Adherence to ketogenic dietary therapies in epilepsy: A systematic review of literature.*". Nutrition Research.

Netzer, N. C. (2024). "*Influence of nutrition and food on sleep—is there evidence?.*". Sleep and Breathing.

Neugut, A. I. (2016). "*Nonadherence to medications for chronic conditions and nonadherence to adjuvant hormonal therapy in women with breast cancer.*". JAMA oncology.

Neuhouser, M. L. (2008). "*Use of recovery biomarkers to calibrate nutrient consumption self-reports in the Women's Health Initiative.*". American journal of epidemiology.

Nguyen, M.-K. e. (2023). "*Occurrence, fate, and potential risk of pharmaceutical pollutants in agriculture: Challenges and environmentally friendly solutions.*". Science of The Total Environment.

Nichele, S. S. (2022). "*Plant-based food patterns to stimulate muscle protein synthesis and support muscle mass in humans: A narrative review.*". Applied Physiology, Nutrition, and Metabolism.

Nickel, K. B. (2022). *Individualized risk prediction tool for serious wound complications after mastectomy with and without immediate reconstruction.* Annals of surgical oncology.

Nijholt, W. e. (2017). "*The reliability and validity of ultrasound to quantify muscles in older adults: a systematic review.*". Journal of cachexia, sarcopenia and muscle.

Nilsson, S. e. (2022). "*Resistance training reduced luteinising hormone levels in postmenopausal women in a substudy of a randomised controlled clinical trial: A clue to how resistance training reduced vasomotor symptoms.*". Plos one.

Nindita, Y. e. (2023). *"Population-Based Impact of Smoking, Drinking, and Genetic Factors on HDL-cholesterol Levels in J-MICC Study Participants."*. Journal of epidemiology.

Nino de Guzman, E. e. (2020). *"Healthcare providers' adherence to breast cancer guidelines in Europe: a systematic literature review."*. Breast cancer research and treatment.

Nissensohn, M. e. (2016). *The effect of the Mediterranean diet on hypertension: a systematic review and meta-analysis."*. Journal of Nutrition Education and Behavior.

Niu, S.-F. e. (2011). *"The effect of shift rotation on employee cortisol profile, sleep quality, fatigue, and attention level: a systematic review."*. Journal of Nursing Research.

Noba, L. a. (2019). *"Are carbohydrate drinks more effective than preoperative fasting: a systematic review of randomised controlled trials."*. Journal of clinical nursing.

Noba, L. e. (2023). *"Costs and clinical benefits of enhanced recovery after surgery (ERAS) in pancreaticoduodenectomy: an updated systematic review and meta-analysis."*. Journal of Cancer Research and Clinical Oncology.

Nolan, M. e. (2019). *"Design, implementation, and evaluation of an intervention to improve referral to smoking cessation services in breast cancer patients."*. Supportive Care in Cancer.

Norman, K. e. (2015). *"The bioimpedance phase angle predicts low muscle strength, impaired quality of life, and increased mortality in old patients with cancer."*. Journal of the American Medical Directors Association.

Norton, D. W. (2024). *"Sleep disturbance mediates the link between both self-compassion and self-criticism and psychological distress during prolonged periods of stress."*. Applied Psychology: Health and Well-Being.

Novara, C. e. (2022). *"The role of dieting, psychopathological characteristics and maladaptive personality traits in Orthorexia Nervosa."*. BMC psychiatry.

Novelle, M. G. (2018). *"Food addiction and binge eating: lessons learned from animal models."*. Nutrients.

Novelle, M. G. (2021). *"Decoding the role of gut-microbiome in the food addiction paradigm."*. International Journal of Environmental Research and Public Health.

Nuñez de Arenas-Arroyo, S. e. (2023). *"Effects of exercise interventions to reduce chemotherapy-induced peripheral neuropathy severity: a meta-analysis."*. Scandinavian Journal of Medicine & Science in Sports.

Oberguggenberger, A. e. (2018). *"Health behavior and quality of life outcome in breast cancer survivors: prevalence rates and predictors."*. Clinical breast cancer.

O'Donnell, M. J. (2016). *"Global and regional effects of potentially modifiable risk factors associated with acute stroke in 32 countries (INTERSTROKE): a case-control study."*. The lancet.

Offodile, A. C. (2019). *"Enhanced recovery after surgery (ERAS) pathways in breast reconstruction: systematic review and meta-analysis of the literature."*. Breast cancer research and treatment.

Ogilvie, A. R. (2022). *"Fracture Risk in Vegetarians and Vegans: The Role of Diet and Metabolic Factors."*. Current osteoporosis reports.

Ohlau, M. A. (2022). *"Plant-based diets are not enough? Understanding the consumption of plant-based meat alternatives along ultra-processed foods in different dietary patterns in Germany."*. Frontiers in nutrition.

O'Connor, K. L. (2016). *"Altered appetite-mediating hormone concentrations precede compensatory overeating after severe, short-term energy deprivation in healthy adults."*. The Journal of nutrition.

Okorodudu, D. O. (2010). *"Diagnostic performance of body mass index to identify obesity as defined by body adiposity: a systematic review and meta-analysis."*. International journal of obesity.

Opoku, A. A. (2023). *"Obesity and menopause."* . Best Practice & Research Clinical Obstetrics & Gynaecology.

Orscelik, A. G. (2023). *"The relationship of exercise addiction with alexithymia and orthorexia."*. Spor Hekimliği Dergisi.

Ortega, J. F. (2015). *"Higher insulin-sensitizing response after sprint interval compared to continuous exercise."*. International journal of sports medicine.

Osman, M. A. (2015). *Obesity correlation with metastases development and response to first-line metastatic chemotherapy in breast cancer.* Clinical Medicine Insights: Oncology.

Oxfeldt, M. e. (2023). *"Low energy availability reduces myofibrillar and sarcoplasmic muscle protein synthesis in trained females."*. The Journal of Physiology.

Padilha, C. S. (2017). *"Evaluation of resistance training to improve muscular strength and body composition in cancer patients undergoing neoadjuvant and adjuvant therapy: a meta-analysis."*. Journal of Cancer Survivorship.

Palmer, K. e. (2018). *"The relationship between anaemia and frailty: a systematic review and meta-analysis of observational studies."*. The Journal of nutrition, health and aging.

Pamoukdjian, F. e. (2018). *"Prevalence and predictive value of pre-therapeutic sarcopenia in cancer patients: a systematic review."*. Clinical Nutrition.

Panayi, A. C. (2018). *Impact of obesity on outcomes in breast reconstruction: a systematic review and meta-analysis.* Journal of reconstructive microsurgery.

Pang, Y. Y. (2022). *"Associations of adiposity and weight change with recurrence and survival in breast cancer patients: a systematic review and meta-analysis."*. Breast cancer.

Paoli, A. e. (2015). *"Ketosis, ketogenic diet and food intake control: a complex relationship."*. Frontiers in psychology.

Paoli, A. e. (2023). *"The effects of ketogenic diet on insulin sensitivity and weight loss, which came first: the chicken or the egg?."*. Nutrients.

Papadopetraki, A. e. (2023). *"The role of exercise in cancer-related sarcopenia and sarcopenic obesity."*. Cancers.

Pappa, S. N. (2022). *"A year in review: sleep dysfunction and psychological distress in healthcare workers during the COVID-19 pandemic."*. Sleep medicine.

Paranjpe, R. e. (2019). *"Identifying adherence barriers to oral endocrine therapy among breast cancer survivors."*. Breast Cancer Research and Treatment.

Parikh, S. J. (2004). *The relationship between obesity and serum 1, 25-dihydroxy vitamin D concentrations in healthy adults*. The Journal of Clinical Endocrinology & Metabolism.

Park, S.-H. M. (2019). *"Endocrine therapy–related symptoms and quality of life in female cancer survivors in the Yale Fitness Intervention Trial."*. Journal of Nursing Scholarship.

Park, S.-A. e. (2010). *Normal physiologic and benign foci with F-18 FDG avidity on PET/CT in patients with breast cancer*. Nuclear medicine and molecular imaging.

Park, Y.-M. M. (2017). *The association between metabolic health, obesity phenotype and the risk of breast cancer*. International journal of cancer.

Parker, J. J. (2017). *Risk factors for the development of acute radiation dermatitis in breast cancer patients*. International Journal of Radiation Oncology, Biology, Physics.

Parmenter, B. H. (2017). *"Accuracy and precision of estimation equations to predict net endogenous acid excretion using the Australian food database."*. Nutrition & dietetics.

Parmenter, B. H. (2020). *"Performance of predictive equations and biochemical measures quantifying net endogenous acid production and the potential renal acid load."*. Kidney International Reports.

Parodi, P. W. (2007). *"A role for milk proteins and their peptides in cancer prevention."*. Current pharmaceutical design.

Parry, S. A. (2017). *"A single day of excessive dietary fat intake reduces whole-body insulin sensitivity: the metabolic consequence of binge eating."* . Nutrients.

Passarelli, M. N. (2016). *"Cigarette smoking before and after breast cancer diagnosis: mortality from breast cancer and smoking-related diseases."*. Journal of Clinical Oncology.

Pataka, A. e. (2022). *"Sleep disorders and mental stress of healthcare workers during the two first waves of COVID-19 pandemic: separate analysis for primary care."*. Healthcare.

Patel, S. e. (2015). *"Alcohol and the Intestine."*. Biomolecules.

Patel, V. e. (2020). *"Body mass index and outcomes in breast cancer treated with breast conservation."*. International Journal of Radiation Oncology* Biology* Physics.

Paterson, C. L. (2016). *"Body image in younger breast cancer survivors: a systematic review."*. Cancer nursing.

Pavlides, S. e. (2009). *The reverse Warburg effect: aerobic glycolysis in cancer associated fibroblasts and the tumor stroma.* Cell cycle.

Pavlovic, D. e. (2023). *"CDK4/6 inhibitors: basics, pros, and major cons in breast cancer treatment with specific regard to cardiotoxicity–a narrative review."*. Therapeutic Advances in Medical Oncology.

Pawlak, R. J. (2018). *"Iron status of vegetarian adults: a review of literature."*. American journal of lifestyle medicine.

Pearson, O. e. (2023). *"The relationship between sleep disturbance and cognitive impairment in mood disorders: A systematic review."*. Journal of affective disorders.

Pedroso, C. M. (2023). *"Pan-American prevalence of smokeless tobacco use and association with oral potentially malignant disorders and head and neck cancer: a systematic review and meta-analysis."*. Oral Surgery, Oral Medicine, Oral Pathology and Oral Radiology.

Pender, K. D. (2023). *"Preserving choice in breast cancer treatment: A different perspective on contralateral prophylactic mastectomy."*. Women's Health.

Pereira, M. M. (2018). *"The prognostic role of phase angle in advanced cancer patients: a systematic review."*. Nutrition in Clinical Practice.

Pérez-Bilbao, T. e. (2023). *"Effects of combined interventions of exercise and diet or exercise and supplementation on breast cancer patients: A systematic review."*. Nutrients.

Petersen, J. M. (2021). *"A systematic review of quantitative bias analysis applied to epidemiological research."*. International journal of epidemiology.

Petersson, M. e. (2017). *"Oxytocin and cortisol levels in dog owners and their dogs are associated with behavioral patterns: An exploratory study."*. Frontiers in psychology.

Petito, E. L. (2014). *The influence of the initiation of an exercise programme on seroma formation and dehiscence following breast cancer surgery.* Journal of clinical nursing.

Petrakis, N. L. (1996). *"Stimulatory influence of soy protein isolate on breast secretion in pre-and postmenopausal women."*. Cancer epidemiology, biomarkers & prevention: a publication of the American Association for Cancer Research, cosponsored by the American Society of Preventive Oncology.

Petri, A. L. (2004). *"Alcohol intake, type of beverage, and risk of breast cancer in pre-and postmenopausal women."*. Alcoholism: Clinical and Experimental Research.

Petroni, M. L. (2019). *"Moderate alcohol intake in non-alcoholic fatty liver disease: to drink or not to drink?."*. Nutrients.

Petry, N. (2014). *"Polyphenols and low iron bioavailability."*. Polyphenols in human health and disease.

Pierobon, M. a. (2013). *Obesity as a risk factor for triple-negative breast cancers: a systematic review and meta-analysis.* Breast cancer research and treatment.

Pilkington, P. D. (2024). *"Early maladaptive schemas, emotion regulation difficulties and alexithymia: A systematic review and meta-analysis."*. Clinical Psychology & Psychotherapy.

Pinckaers, P. J. (2023). *"Higher muscle protein synthesis rates following ingestion of an omnivorous meal compared with an isocaloric and isonitrogenous vegan meal in healthy, older adults."*. The Journal of nutrition.

Pittelkow, E. M. (2020). *"Preoperatively identified sarcopenia leads to increased postoperative complications, hospital and ICU length of stay in autologous microsurgical breast reconstruction."*. Journal of Reconstructive Microsurgery.

Pizzuti, L. e. (2017). *"Anthropometric, clinical and molecular determinants of treatment outcomes in postmenopausal, hormone receptor positive metastatic breast cancer patients treated with fulvestrant: Results from a real word setting."*. Oncotarget.

Planas, M. e. (2016). *"Prevalence of hospital malnutrition in cancer patients: a sub-analysis of the PREDyCES® study."*. Supportive Care in Cancer.

Playdon, M. C. (2015). *"Weight gain after breast cancer diagnosis and all-cause mortality: systematic review and meta-analysis."*. Journal of the National Cancer Institute.

Playdon, M. C. (2015). *Weight gain after breast cancer diagnosis and all-cause mortality: systematic review and meta-analysis.* Journal of the National Cancer Institute.

Pokala, A. e. (2024). "*Whole-Milk Dairy Foods and Cardiometabolic Health: Dairy Fat and Beyond.*". Nutrition Research.

Polk, A. e. (2016). "*Incidence and risk factors for capecitabine-induced symptomatic cardiotoxicity: a retrospective study of 452 consecutive patients with metastatic breast cancer.*". Bmj Open.

Posadzki, P. L. (2013). "*Adverse effects of herbal medicines: an overview of systematic reviews.*". Clinical medicine.

Prado, C. M. (2020). *Nutrition interventions to treat low muscle mass in cancer.* Journal of cachexia, sarcopenia and muscle.

Prentice, R. L. (2006). "*Low-fat dietary pattern and risk of invasive breast cancer: the Women's Health Initiative Randomized Controlled Dietary Modification Trial.*". Jama.

Prochaska, J. O. (1991). "*Assessing how people change.*". Cancer.

Prokopidis, K. e. (2023). "*Sarcopenia is associated with a greater risk of polypharmacy and number of medications: a systematic review and meta-analysis.*". Journal of cachexia, sarcopenia and muscle.

Protani, M. M. (2010). *Effect of obesity on survival of women with breast cancer: systematic review and meta-analysis.* Breast cancer research and treatment.

Purchas, R. W. (2003). "*Variation in the form of iron in beef and lamb meat and losses of iron during cooking and storage.*". International journal of food science & technology.

Qian, W. e. (2014). "*Decreased circulating levels of oxytocin in obesity and newly diagnosed type 2 diabetic patients.*". The Journal of Clinical Endocrinology & Metabolism.

Qin, G.-Q. e. (2023). "*Effect of passive smoking exposure on risk of type 2 diabetes: a systematic review and meta-analysis of prospective cohort studies.*". Frontiers in Endocrinology.

Qin, Y. e. (2023). "*Autophagy and cancer drug resistance in dialogue: pre-clinical and clinical evidence.*". Cancer letters.

Quartiroli, M. e. (2024). "*Adherence to Diet Quality Indices and Breast Cancer Risk in the Italian ORDET Cohort.*". Nutrients.

Quesnel, D. A. (2023). *"Medical and physiological complications of exercise for individuals with an eating disorder: A narrative review."*. Journal of Eating Disorders.

Quinn, D. M. (2020). *"Trying again (and again): Weight cycling and depressive symptoms in US adults."*. Plos one.

Römer, M. J. (2021). *"The use of ketogenic diets in cancer patients: a systematic review."*. Clinical and experimental medicine.

Rüggeberg, A. P. (2024). *"Preoperative fasting and the risk of pulmonary aspiration—a narrative review of historical concepts, physiological effects, and new perspectives."*. BJA open.

Rabelo, A. C. (2024). *"The Role of Soy and Its Isoflavones in Breast Cancer: Beneficial or Harmful?."*. Springer.

Raichur, S. R. (2017). *"Correlation of serum ferritin levels, in female patients with chronic diffuse hair loss: A cross sectional study."*. Indian Journal of Health Sciences and Biomedical Research.

Rajan, K. K. (2024). *"Overall survival after mastectomy versus breast-conserving surgery with adjuvant radiotherapy for early-stage breast cancer: meta-analysis."*. BJS open.

Rajaram, N. N. (2022). *A causal investigation of soy isoflavone intake for primary prevention of post-menopausal breast cancer among Asian women.* Diss. University of Nottingham.

Ramírez-Vélez, R. e. (2021). *"Effect of exercise on myosteatosis in adults: a systematic review and meta-analysis."*. Journal of Applied Physiology.

Raninen, J. e. (2023). *"Trends in Tobacco Use among 9th Graders in Sweden, 1991–2020."*. nternational Journal of Environmental Research and Public Health.

Ranjbar, S. e. (2017). *"Emerging roles of probiotics in prevention and treatment of breast cancer: a comprehensive review of their therapeutic potential."*. Nutrition and cancer.

Ranjbar, S. e. (2019). *"Emerging roles of probiotics in prevention and treatment of breast cancer: a comprehensive review of their therapeutic potential."*. Nutrition and cancer.

Rantakömi, S. H. (2013). *"Alcohol consumption and the risk of stroke among hypertensive and overweight men."*. Journal of neurology.

Rasschaert, M. e. (2024). *"Malnutrition prevalence in cancer patients in Belgium: The ONCOCARE study."*. Supportive Care in Cancer.

Rassool, G. H. (2011). *Understanding addiction behaviours: Theoretical and clinical practice in health and social care.* Bloomsbury Publishing.

Ratosa, I. A. (2018). *"Breast size impact on adjuvant radiotherapy adverse effects and dose parameters in treatment planning.""Breast size impact on adjuvant radiotherapy adverse effects and dose parameters in treatment planning."*. Radiology and oncology.

Rees, K. e. (2019). *"Mediterranean-style diet for the primary and secondary prevention of cardiovascular disease."*. Cochrane Database of Systematic Reviews.

Reis, A. R. (2023). *"Supplementation of vitamin D isolated or calcium-associated with bone remodeling and fracture risk in postmenopausal women without osteoporosis: A systematic review of randomized clinical trials."*. Nutrition.

Rezaianzadeh, A. e. (2018). *"Red meat consumption and breast cancer risk in premenopausal women: A systematic review and meta-analysis."*. Middle East Journal of Cancer.

Ricci-Cabello, I. e. (2020). *"Adherence to breast cancer guidelines is associated with better survival outcomes: a systematic review and meta-analysis of observational studies in EU countries."*. BMC health services research.

Rich, M. D. (2022). *"Routine Preoperative Nutritional Optimization Not Required in Patients Undergoing Breast Reconstruction."*. Breast Care.

Richardson, H. a. (2012). *"The Goldilocks mastectomy"*. International Journal of Surgery.

Richter, C. P. (1941). *"Behavior and endocrine regulators of the internal environment."*. Endocrinology.

Richter, M. e. (2016). *"Vegan diet. Position of the German nutrition society (DGE)."*. Ernahrungs umschau.

Ring, T. a. (2017). *"Whole body acid-base modeling revisited."*. American Journal of Physiology-Renal Physiology.

Roberto, M. e. (2024). *"Sarcopenia in Breast Cancer Patients: A Systematic Review and Meta-Analysis."*. Cancers.

Robertson, R. P. (2023). *"Brief overview: glucagon history and physiology."*. Journal of Endocrinology.

Robinson, P. J. (2014). *Obesity is associated with a poorer prognosis in women with hormone receptor positive breast cancer.* Maturitas.

Rock, C. L. (2000). *"Eating pathology and obesity in women at risk for breast cancer recurrence."*. International Journal of Eating Disorders.

Rodgers, G. M. (2012). *"Cancer-and chemotherapy-induced anemia."*. Journal of the National Comprehensive Cancer Network.

Rodgers, K. M. (2017). *Environmental pollutants and breast cancer: 2006-2016 epidemiological studies designed to evaluate biological hypotheses provide evidence of risk for certain pesticides, organic solvents, and products of combustion.* Cancer Research.

Rodin, J. (1985). *"Insulin levels, hunger, and food intake: an example of feedback loops in body weight regulation."*. Health Psychology.

Rodríguez-Alcalá, L. M. (2017). *"Milk fat components with potential anticancer activity—a review."*. Bioscience reports.

Rohrmann, S. e. (2015). *"Meat and fish consumption and the risk of renal cell carcinoma in the E uropean prospective investigation into cancer and nutrition."*. International journal of cancer.

Rojas, K. e. (2023). *"Endocrine Therapy for Surgeons: Practical Pearls for Managing Menopausal, Bone Loss and Sexual Adverse Effects."*. Annals of surgical oncology.

Romero-Corral, A. e. (2008). *"Accuracy of body mass index in diagnosing obesity in the adult general population."*. International journal of obesity.

Romo, L. e. (2024). *"A Qualitative Model of Weight Cycling."*. Qualitative Health Research.

Ronis, M. J. (2018). *"Adverse effects of nutraceuticals and dietary supplements."*. Annual review of pharmacology and toxicology.

Ronksley, P. E. (2011). *"Association of alcohol consumption with selected cardiovascular disease outcomes: a systematic review and meta-analysis."*. Bmj.

Rosenman, R. H. (1970). *"Coronary heart disease in the Western Collaborative Group Study: A follow-up experience of 412 years."*. Journal of Chronic Diseases.

Rossi, F. e. (2019). *"Evaluation of body computed tomography-determined sarcopenia in breast cancer patients and clinical outcomes: a systematic review."*. Cancer Treatment and Research Communications.

Rossi, F. e. (2023). *"Muscle mass loss in breast cancer patients of reproductive age (≤ 45 years) undergoing neoadjuvant chemotherapy."*. La radiologia medica.

Rota, M. e. (2024). *"Dose–response association between cigarette smoking and gastric cancer risk: a systematic review and meta-analysis."*. Gastric Cancer.

Roumeliotis, G. A. (2017). *"Complementary and alternative medicines and patients with breast cancer: a case of mortality and systematic review of patterns of use in patients with breast cancer."*. Plastic Surgery.

Rudzińska, A. e. (2023). *"Phytochemicals in cancer treatment and cancer prevention—review on epidemiological data and clinical trials."*. Nutrients.

Rudzińska, A. e. (2023). *"Phytochemicals in cancer treatment and cancer prevention—review on epidemiological data and clinical trials."*. Nutrients.

Ruggiero, J. S. (2014). *"Effects of napping on sleepiness and sleep-related performance deficits in night-shift workers: a systematic review."*. Biological research for nursing.

Rugo, H. S. (2023). *"Real-world perspectives and practices for pneumonitis/interstitial lung disease associated with trastuzumab deruxtecan use in human epidermal growth factor receptor 2–expressing metastatic breast cancer."*. JCO oncology practice.

Rumawas, M. E. (2009). *"The development of the Mediterranean-style dietary pattern score and its application to the American diet in the Framingham Offspring Cohort."*. The Journal of nutrition.

Rumgay, H. e. (2021). *Global burden of cancer in 2020 attributable to alcohol consumption: a population-based study."*. The Lancet Oncology.

Sørensen, L. T. (2002). *"Smoking as a risk factor for wound healing and infection in breast cancer surgery."*. European Journal of Surgical Oncology.

Sørensen, M. e. (2014). *Exposure to road traffic and railway noise and postmenopausal breast cancer: a cohort study.* International journal of cancer.

Sabiston, C. M. (2012). *Pain, movement, and mind: does physical activity mediate the relationship between pain and mental health among survivors of breast cancer?* The Clinical journal of pain.

Sabitovic, A. H. (2023). *"The impact of neoadjuvant chemotherapy on surgical outcomes following autologous and implant-based immediate breast reconstruction: A systematic review and meta-analysis."*. Journal of Plastic, Reconstructive & Aesthetic Surgery.

Sabol, R. A. (2020). *"Obesity-altered adipose stem cells promote radiation resistance of estrogen receptor positive breast cancer through paracrine signaling."*. International journal of molecular sciences.

Sachdeva, S. R. (2009). *"Sinning saints and saintly sinners: The paradox of moral self-regulation."*. Psychological science.

Sachs, B. D. (2013). *"The effects of brain serotonin deficiency on behavioural disinhibition and anxiety-like behaviour following mild early life stress."*. International Journal of Neuropsychopharmacology.

Sadeghirad, B. e. (2014). *"Islamic fasting and weight loss: a systematic review and meta-analysis."*. Public health nutrition.

Sadok, N. e. (2022). *"The effect of sarcopenic obesity and muscle quality on complications after DIEP-flap breast reconstruction."*. Heliyon.

Said Abasse, K. e. (2022). *"Association between dietary nitrate, nitrite intake, and site-specific cancer risk: a systematic review and meta-analysis."*. Nutrients.

Salerno, E. A. (2021). *"Physical activity patterns and relationships with cognitive function in patients with breast cancer before, during, and after chemotherapy in a prospective, nationwide study."*. Journal of Clinical Oncology.

Sallie, S. N. (2020). *"Assessing international alcohol consumption patterns during isolation from the COVID-19 pandemic using an online survey: highlighting negative emotionality mechanisms."*. BMJ open.

Sanaya, N. e. (2024). *"The Physiological Effects of Weight-Cycling: A Review of Current Evidence."*. Current Obesity Reports.

Sanchez-Rodriguez, D. E.-J. (2020). *"Defining sarcopenia: some caveats and challenges."* . Current Opinion in Clinical Nutrition & Metabolic Care.

Sanchez-Villegas, A. e. (2006). *"Adherence to a Mediterranean dietary pattern and weight gain in a follow-up study: the SUN cohort."*. International journal of obesity.

Sanford, N. N. (2020). *"Alcohol use among patients with cancer and survivors in the United States, 2000–2017."*. Journal of the National Comprehensive Cancer Network.

Santos, W. D. (2019). *"Once a week resistance training improves muscular strength in breast cancer survivors: a randomized controlled trial."*. Integrative cancer therapies.

Saraf, A. e. (2024). *"Association of Sarcopenia With Toxicity-Related Discontinuation of Adjuvant Endocrine Therapy in Women With Early-Stage Hormone Receptor–Positive Breast Cancer."*. International Journal of Radiation Oncology* Biology* Physics.

Sarhane, K. A. (2013). *"Preoperative anemia and postoperative outcomes in immediate breast reconstructive surgery: a critical analysis of 10,958 patients from the ACS-NSQIP database."*. Plastic and Reconstructive Surgery–Global Open.

Sarhane, K. A. (2013). *"Preoperative anemia and postoperative outcomes in immediate breast reconstructive surgery: a critical analysis of 10,958 patients from the ACS-NSQIP database."*. Plastic and Reconstructive Surgery–Global Open.

Sartippour, M. R. (2004). *"A pilot clinical study of short-term isoflavone supplements in breast cancer patients."*. Nutrition and cancer.

Sauder, C. A. (2020). *"Breast conserving surgery compared with mastectomy in male breast cancer: a brief systematic review."*. Clinical breast cancer.

Saules, K. K. (2018). *"Overeating, overweight, and substance use: what is the connection?."*. Current Addiction Reports.

Savaiano, D. A. (2021). *"Yogurt, cultured fermented milk, and health: A systematic review."*. Nutrition reviews.

Savaiano, D. A. (2021). *"Yogurt, cultured fermented milk, and health: A systematic review."*. Nutrition reviews.

Savard, J. e. (2009). *"Breast cancer patients have progressively impaired sleep-wake activity rhythms during chemotherapy."*. Sleep.

Savelberg, W. e. (2019). *"Does lack of deeper understanding of shared decision making explains the suboptimal performance on crucial parts of it? An example from breast cancer care."*. European Journal of Oncology Nursing.

Savelberg, W. e. (2019). *"Does lack of deeper understanding of shared decision making explains the suboptimal performance on crucial parts of it? An example from breast cancer care."*. European Journal of Oncology Nursing.

Sayuk, G. S. (2023). *"Management of Constipation in Hospitalized Patients."*. Journal of Clinical Medicine.

Scala, M. e. (2023). *"Dose-response relationships between cigarette smoking and breast cancer risk: a systematic review and meta-analysis."*. Journal of Epidemiology.

Schaverien, M. V. (2014). *Effect of obesity on outcomes of free autologous breast reconstruction: A meta-analysis.* Microsurgery.

Schlesinger, S. e. (2017). *"Carbohydrates, glycemic index, glycemic load, and breast cancer risk: a systematic review and dose–response meta-analysis of prospective studies."*. Nutrition reviews.

Schmid, D. a. (2014). *Television viewing and time spent sedentary in relation to cancer risk: a meta-analysis.* Journal of the National Cancer Institute.

Schmid, S. M. (2012). *"Impact of body mass index on compliance and persistence to adjuvant breast cancer therapy."*. The Breast.

Schreiber, K. L. (2014). *"Predicting, preventing and managing persistent pain after breast cancer surgery: the importance of psychosocial factors."*. Pain management .

Schuchmann, S. e. (2011). *"Respiratory alkalosis in children with febrile seizures."*. Epilepsia.

Schwingshackl, L. a. (2014). *"Adherence to Mediterranean diet and risk of cancer: a systematic review and meta-analysis of observational studies."*. International journal of cancer.

Schwingshackl, L. e. (2015). *"Adherence to a Mediterranean diet and risk of diabetes: a systematic review and meta-analysis."*. Public health nutrition.

Schwingshackl, L. e. (2017). *"Adherence to Mediterranean diet and risk of cancer: an updated systematic review and meta-analysis."*. Nutrients.

Scialla, J. J. (2017). *"Higher net acid excretion is associated with a lower risk of kidney disease progression in patients with diabetes."*. Kidney international.

Secretan, B. e. (2009). *A review of human carcinogens—Part E: tobacco, areca nut, alcohol, coal smoke, and salted fish."*. The lancet oncology.

Seitz, H. K. (2012). *"Epidemiology and pathophysiology of alcohol and breast cancer: Update 2012."*. Alcohol and alcoholism.

Seitz, H. K. (2015). *"Effect of chronic alcohol consumption on the development and progression of non-alcoholic fatty liver disease (NAFLD)."*. Hepatobiliary surgery and nutrition.

Selçuk, K. T. (2020). *"Use of dietary supplements among nursing students in Turkey in the last 12 months and its relation with orthorexia nervosa."*. Perspectives in Psychiatric Care.

Selinger, E. e. (2023). *"Evidence of a vegan diet for health benefits and risks–an umbrella review of meta-analyses of observational and clinical studies."*. CritiCal reviews in Food sCienCe and nutrition.

Selinger, E. e. (2023). *"Evidence of a vegan diet for health benefits and risks–an umbrella review of meta-analyses of observational and clinical studies."*. CritiCal reviews in Food sCienCe and nutrition.

Selinger, E. e. (2023). *"Evidence of a vegan diet for health benefits and risks–an umbrella review of meta-analyses of observational and clinical studies."*. CritiCal reviews in Food sCienCe and nutrition.

Sella, T. e. (2022). *"Body weight changes and associated predictors in a prospective cohort of young breast cancer survivors."*. Cancer.

Seman, D. L. (2018). *"Meat science lexicon."*. Meat and Muscle Biology.

Sendur, M. A. (2016). *"Effect of body mass index on the efficacy of adjuvant tamoxifen in premenopausal patients with hormone receptor-positive breast cancer."*. J BUON.

Seo, H. S. (2020). *"Changes of neurotransmitters in youth with internet and smartphone addiction: A comparison with healthy controls and changes after cognitive behavioral therapy."*. American Journal of Neuroradiology.

Serio, F. e. (2023). *"Moderate Red Wine Consumption and cardiovascular Health Protection: a literature review."*. Food & Function.

Sestak, I. e. (2010). *"Effect of body mass index on recurrences in tamoxifen and anastrozole treated women: an exploratory analysis from the ATAC trial."*. Journal of Clinical Oncology.

Setchell, K. D. (2003). *"Variations in isoflavone levels in soy foods and soy protein isolates and issues related to isoflavone databases and food labeling."*. Journal of Agricultural and Food Chemistry.

Sfeir, M. e. (2022). *"Association between religiosity and orthorexia nervosa with the mediating role of self-esteem among a sample of the Lebanese population–short communication."*. Journal of Eating Disorders.

Shachar, S. S. (2016). *"Prognostic value of sarcopenia in adults with solid tumours: a meta-analysis and systematic review."*. European journal of cancer.

Shah, A. D. (2016). *"Less favorable body composition and adipokines in South Asians compared with other US ethnic groups: results from the MASALA and MESA studies."*. International journal of obesity.

Sharma, R. a. (2023). *"Global burden of cancers attributable to tobacco smoking, 1990–2019: an ecological study."*. EPMA Journal.

Shea, M. K. (2019). *"Vitamin E: Interactions with Vitamin K and Other Bioactive Compounds."*. Springer: Vitamin E in Human Health.

Shea, M. K. (2019). *"Vitamin E: Interactions with Vitamin K and Other Bioactive Compounds."*. Springer: Vitamin E in Human Health .

Sheean, P. e. (2021). *"Myosteatosis at diagnosis is adversely associated with 2-year survival in women with estrogen receptor-negative metastatic breast cancer."*. Breast Cancer Research and Treatment.

Shen, A. e. (2023). *Risk factors of unilateral breast cancer-related lymphedema: an updated systematic review and meta-analysis of 84 cohort studies.* Supportive Care in Cancer.

Shete, A. V. (2023). *"Safety of E-cigarettes and its effectiveness in smoking cessation: A systematic review."*. Journal of International Oral Health.

Shi, M. e. (2023). *"Alcohol Consumption among Adults with a Cancer Diagnosis in the All of Us Research Program."*. JAMA Network Open.

Shike, M. e. (2014). *"The effects of soy supplementation on gene expression in breast cancer: a randomized placebo-controlled study."*. JNCI: Journal of the National Cancer Institute.

Shin, J. Y. (2016). *"Is obesity a predisposing factor for free flap failure and complications? Comparison between breast and nonbreast reconstruction: Systematic review and meta-analysis."*. Medicine.

Shoaib, M. a. (2018). *"Why are antidepressant drugs effective smoking cessation aids?."*. Current Neuropharmacology.

Shorthouse, D. e. (2022). *"Heterogeneity of the cancer cell line metabolic landscape."*. Molecular Systems Biology.

Shrank, W. H. (2019). *"Waste in the US health care system: estimated costs and potential for savings."*. Jama.

Sierksma, A. e. (2004). *"Effect of moderate alcohol consumption on parameters of reverse cholesterol transport in postmenopausal women."*. Alcoholism: Clinical and Experimental Research.

Silvani, M. I. (2022). *"The influence of blue light on sleep, performance and wellbeing in young adults: A systematic review."*. Frontiers in physiology.

Sim, J.-H. e. (2024). *"Association between Sarcopenia and Survival in Patients Undergoing Gamma Knife Surgery for Brain Metastasis *from Breast Cancer: A Retrospective Single-centre Cohort Study.".* Clinical Oncology.

Simapivapan, P. A. (2016). *"To what extent is alcohol consumption associated with breast cancer recurrence and second primary breast cancer?: A systematic review.".* Cancer Treatment Reviews.

Simon, V. e. (2020). *"No impact of smoking status on breast cancer tumor infiltrating lymphocytes, response to neoadjuvant chemotherapy and prognosis.".* Cancers.

Simpkin, A. (2020). *Burnout in medicine: A novel approach exploring the impact of uncertainty and the use of biomarkers as a measurement tool.* Diss. University of Oxford.

Singh, B. e. (2014). *"Association of mediterranean diet with mild cognitive impairment and Alzheimer's disease: a systematic review and meta-analysis.".* Journal of Alzheimer's disease.

Singh, B. e. (2016). *"Systematic review and meta-analysis of the effects of exercise for those with cancer-related lymphedema.".* Archives of physical medicine and rehabilitation.

Singh, T. e. (2022). *"Does Insufficient Sleep Increase the Risk of Developing Insulin Resistance: A Systematic Review.".* Cureus.

Sinik, L. e. (2022). *"A Systematic Review of Breast Reconstruction Options After Mastectomy in Massive Weight Loss Patients.".* Annals of Plastic Surgery.

Sinik, L. M. (2023). *"Autologous Breast Reconstruction after Massive Weight Loss: Understanding Risks in a Growing Population.".* Plastic and Reconstructive Surgery.

Sletten, T. L. (2023). *"The importance of sleep regularity: a consensus statement of the National Sleep Foundation sleep timing and variability panel.".* Sleep Health.

Slimani, N. e. (2003). *"Group level validation of protein intakes estimated by 24-hour diet recall and dietary questionnaires against 24-hour urinary nitrogen in the European Prospective Investigation into Cancer and Nutrition (EPIC) calibration study.".* Cancer Epidemiology Biomarkers & Prevention.

Smith, M. G. (2022). *"Environmental noise and effects on sleep: an update to the WHO systematic review and meta-analysis.".* Environmental health perspectives.

Smolková, K. e. (2010). *Mitochondrial bioenergetic adaptations of breast cancer cells to aglycemia and hypoxia.* Journal of bioenergetics and biomembranes.

Snoek, A. e. (2021). *"Managing shame and guilt in addiction: A pathway to recovery.".* Addictive behaviors.

Soeters, M. R. (2012). *"The evolutionary benefit of insulin resistance.".* Clinical nutrition.

Sollie, M. a. (2017). *"Smoking and mortality in women diagnosed with breast cancer—a systematic review with meta-analysis based on 400,944 breast cancer cases.".* Gland surgery.

Sonagli, M. e. (2021). *Postoperative complications following simultaneous therapeutic and contralateral prophylactic nipple-sparing mastectomy: a retrospective study.* Mastology.

Sondrup, N. e. (2022). *"Effects of sleep manipulation on markers of insulin sensitivity: A systematic review and meta-analysis of randomized controlled trials.".* Sleep Medicine Reviews.

Spaggiari, G. e. (2020). *"To beer or not to beer: A meta-analysis of the effects of beer consumption on cardiovascular health."* . PLoS One.

Sparano, J. A. (2012). *Obesity at diagnosis is associated with inferior outcomes in hormone receptor-positive operable breast cancer.* Cancer.

Sprajcer, M. e. (2023). *"How tired is too tired to drive? A systematic review assessing the use of prior sleep duration to detect driving impairment.".* Nature and science of sleep.

Spring, B. e. (2009). *"Behavioral intervention to promote smoking cessation and prevent weight gain: a systematic review and meta-analysis.".* Addiction.

Spring, B. e. (2009). *"Behavioral intervention to promote smoking cessation and prevent weight gain: a systematic review and meta-analysis.".* Addiction.

Stasi, C. S. (2019). *"The relationship between the serotonin metabolism, gut-microbiota and the gut-brain axis.".* Current drug metabolism.

Stefanaki, C. e. (2023). *"Chronic Stress and Steatosis of Muscles, Bones, Liver, and Pancreas: A Review.".* Hormone Research in Paediatrics.

Stephenson Babatunde Ojeifo, M. B. (2018). *Birth-weight and Risk of Breast Cancer: A Systematic Review Study.* Breast cancer.

Stickel, F. a. (2015). *"Hepatotoxicity of herbal and dietary supplements: an update."*. Archives of toxicology.

Stoica, M. e. (2022). *"New strategies for the total/partial replacement of conventional sodium nitrite in meat products: A review."*. Food and Bioprocess Technology.

Stote, K. S. (2016). *"The effect of moderate alcohol consumption on biomarkers of inflammation and hemostatic factors in postmenopausal women."*. European Journal of Clinical Nutrition.

Stout, N. L. (2021). *"A systematic review of rehabilitation and exercise recommendations in oncology guidelines."*. CA: a cancer journal for clinicians.

Strahler, J. (2019). *"Sex differences in orthorexic eating behaviors: A systematic review and meta-analytical integration."*. Nutrition.

Strahler, J. e. (2020). *"Cross-cultural differences in orthorexic eating behaviors: Associations with personality traits."*. Nutrition.

Strong, A. L. (2015). *Leptin produced by obese adipose stromal/stem cells enhances proliferation and metastasis of estrogen receptor positive breast cancers.* Breast Cancer Research.

Stunkard, A. J. (1955). *"The mechanism of satiety: effect of glucagon on gastric hunger contractions in man."*. Proceedings of the Society for Experimental Biology and Medicine.

Su, Y. e. (2024). *"Sarcopenia among treated cancer patients before and after neoadjuvant chemotherapy: a systematic review and meta-analysis of high-quality studies."*. Clinical and Translational Oncology.

Suares, N. C. (2011). *"Systematic review: the effects of fibre in the management of chronic idiopathic constipation."*. Alimentary pharmacology & therapeutics.

Sucholeiki, R. L. (2024). *"Intermittent fasting and its impact on toxicities, symptoms and quality of life in patients on active cancer treatment."*. Cancer Treatment Reviews.

Sun, H. e. (2017). *Triple-negative breast cancer and its association with obesity.* Molecular and clinical oncology.

Sun, M. e. (2018). *"Meta-analysis on shift work and risks of specific obesity types."*. Obesity reviews.

Sun, Q. e. (2020). *"Alcohol consumption by beverage type and risk of breast cancer: a dose-response meta-analysis of prospective cohort studies."*. Alcohol and Alcoholism.

Sundgot-Borgen, J. (2012). *"Are under-and overweight female elite athletes thin and fat? A controlled study."*. Medicine and Science in Sports and Exercise.

Suppli, M. P. (2024). *"Signs of Glucagon Resistance After a 2-Week Hypercaloric Diet Intervention."*. The Journal of Clinical Endocrinology & Metabolism.

Suryanegara, F. D. (2022). *"PCR268 The Impact of Radiotherapy Non-Compliance on the Recurrence and Mortality of Breast Cancer Patients: A Systematic Review."*. Value in Health.

Suryanegara, F. D. (2022). *"PCR268 The Impact of Radiotherapy Non-Compliance on the Recurrence and Mortality of Breast Cancer Patients: A Systematic Review."*. Value in Health.

Svoboda DO, G. H. (1966). *"Aflatoxin B1 injury in rat and monkey liver."*. The American Journal of Pathology.

Swierczynski, J. A. (2014). *Role of abnormal lipid metabolism in development, progression, diagnosis and therapy of pancreatic cancer.* World journal of gastroenterology.

Szendi, K. e. (2024). *"Methodological Challenges and Confounders in Research on the Effects of Ketogenic Diets: A Literature Review of Meta-Analyses.* Foods.

Szymanska, M. e. (2017). *"Psychophysiological effects of oxytocin on parent–child interactions: A literature review on oxytocin and parent–child interactions."*. Psychiatry and Clinical Neurosciences.

Tähkämö, L. T.-K. (2019). *"Systematic review of light exposure impact on human circadian rhythm."*. Chronobiology international.

Tabak, B. A. (2022). *"Social anxiety is associated with greater peripheral oxytocin reactivity to psychosocial stress."*. Psychoneuroendocrinology.

Tagliabue, A. e. (2024). *"Ketogenic diet for epilepsy and obesity: Is it the same?"*. Nutrition, Metabolism and Cardiovascular Diseases.

Tan, K. C. (2004). *"Appropriate body-mass index for Asian populations and its implications for policy and intervention strategies."*. The Lancet.

Tang, S.-c. (2012). *"Effect of soy isoflavones on breast cancer risk among pre-and post-menopausal women: a systematic review of randomized controlled trials."*. HKU Theses Online.

Tang, S.-c. (2012). *"Effect of soy isoflavones on breast cancer risk among pre-and post-menopausal women: a systematic review of randomized controlled trials."*. HKU Theses Online (HKUTO).

Tannen, A. a. (2013). *"Malnutrition in Austrian hospital patients. Prevalence, risk factors, nursing interventions, and quality indicators: a descriptive multicentre study."*. Journal of advanced nursing.

Tappy, L. (2017). *"Health implications of fructose consumption in humans."*. Springer International Publishing.

Taylor, C. e. (2017). *"Estimating the risks of breast cancer radiotherapy: evidence from modern radiation doses to the lungs and heart and from previous randomized trials."*. Journal of Clinical Oncology.

Taylor, G. e. (2014). *"Change in mental health after smoking cessation: systematic review and meta-analysis."*. Bmj.

Taylor, P. N. (2018). *"A review of the growing risk of vitamin D toxicity from inappropriate practice."*. British journal of clinical pharmacology.

Teicholz, N. (2023). *"A short history of saturated fat: the making and unmaking of a scientific consensus."*. Current Opinion in Endocrinology, Diabetes and Obesity.

Temple-Oberle, C. e. (2017). *"Discussion: Consensus review of optimal perioperative care in breast reconstruction: Enhanced Recovery after Surgery (ERAS) Society recommendations."*. Plastic and Reconstructive Surgery.

Templin, T. e. (2019). *"The overweight and obesity transition from the wealthy to the poor in low-and middle-income countries: A survey of household data from 103 countries."*. PLoS medicine.

Tenenbaum, A. R. (2014). *"Hypertriglyceridemia: a too long unfairly neglected major cardiovascular risk factor."*. Cardiovascular diabetology.

Tengland, P.-A. (2012). *"Behavior change or empowerment: on the ethics of health-promotion strategies."*. Public health ethics.

Teodoro, M. C. (2021). *"Grazing's frequency and associations with obesity, psychopathology, and loss of control eating in clinical and community contexts: A systematic review."*. Appetite.

Teras, L. R. (2020). *Sustained weight loss and risk of breast cancer in women 50 years and older: a pooled analysis of prospective data.* JNCI: Journal of the National Cancer Institute.

Termannsen, A.-D. e. (2022). *"Effects of vegan diets on cardiometabolic health: a systematic review and meta-analysis of randomized controlled trials."*. Obesity Reviews.

Termannsen, A.-D. e. (2022). *"Effects of vegan diets on cardiometabolic health: a systematic review and meta-analysis of randomized controlled trials."*. Obesity Reviews.

Thakkar, S. e. (2020). *"Regulatory landscape of dietary supplements and herbal medicines from a global perspective."*. Regulatory Toxicology and Pharmacology.

Tham, S. e. (2020). *"Indoor temperature and health: a global systematic review."*. Public Health.

Thiébaut, A. C. (2007). *"Dietary fat and postmenopausal invasive breast cancer in the National Institutes of Health–AARP Diet and Health Study cohort."*. Journal of the National Cancer Institute.

Thivat, E. e. (2010). *Weight change during chemotherapy changes the prognosis in non metastatic breast cancer for the worse.* BMC cancer.

Thomas, S. J. (2017). *"Sleep, insomnia, and hypertension: current findings and future directions."*. Journal of the American Society of Hypertension.

Thomasset, M. A. (1962). *"Bioelectric properties of tissue. Impedance measurement in clinical medicine. Significance of curves obtained."*. Lyon medical .

Thomson, Z. O. (2017). *Can weight gain be prevented in women receiving treatment for breast cancer? A systematic review of intervention studies.* Obesity Reviews.

Thomson, Z. O. (2017). *Can weight gain be prevented in women receiving treatment for breast cancer? A systematic review of intervention studies.* Obesity reviews.

Thorarinsson, A. e. (2017). *"Patient determinants as independent risk factors for postoperative complications of breast reconstruction."*. Gland surgery.

Thu, M. S. (2023). *"Effect of probiotics in breast cancer: A systematic review and meta-analysis."*. Biology.

Tjønneland, A. e. (2007). *"Alcohol intake and breast cancer risk: the European Prospective Investigation into Cancer and Nutrition (EPIC)."*. Cancer Causes & Control.

Tofthagen, C. e. (2022). *"A systematic review of nutritional lab correlates with chemotherapy induced peripheral neuropathy."*. Journal of Clinical Medicine.

Toivonen, K. I. (2020). *"Potentially modifiable factors associated with adherence to adjuvant endocrine therapy among breast cancer survivors: a systematic review."*. Cancers.

Tong, W. M. (2016). *Obese women experience fewer complications after oncoplastic breast repair following partial mastectomy than after immediate total breast reconstruction.* Plastic and reconstructive surgery.

Tousoulis, D. e. (2008). *"Acute effects of different alcoholic beverages on vascular endothelium, inflammatory markers and thrombosis fibrinolysis system."*. Clinical nutrition.

Traber, M. G.–a.-y.-o. (2008). *Nutrition reviews.* Nutrition reviews.

Tran, B. H. (2013). *"Risk factors associated with venous thromboembolism in 49,028 mastectomy patients."*. The Breast.

Tran, K. a. (2018). *"Intermittent pneumatic compression devices for the management of lymphedema: a review of clinical effectiveness and guidelines."*. Europe PMC.

Trestini, I. e. (2023). *"Predictive and prognostic effect of computed tomography–derived body composition analysis during neoadjuvant chemotherapy for operable and locally advanced breast cancer."*. Nutrition.

Trichopoulou, A. C. (2005). *"Mediterranean diet and survival among patients with coronary heart disease in Greece."*. Archives of Internal Medicine.

Trichopoulou, A. e. (1995). *"Diet and overall survival in elderly people."*. Bmj.

Trieu, K. e. (2021). *"Biomarkers of dairy fat intake, incident cardiovascular disease, and all-cause mortality: A cohort study, systematic review, and meta-analysis."*. PLoS medicine.

Troped, P. J. (2007). *"Reliability and validity of YRBS physical activity items among middle school students."*. Medicine and science in sports and exercise.

Tsai, C.-L. e. (2020). *Effects of weight reduction on the breast cancer-related lymphedema: A systematic review and meta-analysis.* The Breast .

Tsai, Y.-L. e. (2023). *"Feasibility of aerobic exercise training to mitigate cardiotoxicity of breast cancer therapy: a systematic review and meta-analysis."*. Clinical Breast Cancer.

Tsubura, A. e. (2011). *"Anticancer effects of garlic and garlic-derived compounds for breast cancer control."*. Anti-Cancer Agents in Medicinal Chemistry.

Tung, Y.-T. e. (2013). *"Bovine lactoferrin inhibits lung cancer growth through suppression of both inflammation and expression of vascular endothelial growth factor."*. Journal of dairy science.

Turki, S. a. (2012). *"Emerging approaches for the treatment of fat malabsorption due to exocrine pancreatic insufficiency."*. New Advances in the Basic and Clinical Gastroenterology.

Turner, J. A. (2022). *BRAF modulates lipid use and accumulation.* Cancers.

Tzotzas, T. e. (2010). *Rising serum 25-hydroxy-vitamin D levels after weight loss in obese women correlate with improvement in insulin resistance.* The Journal of Clinical Endocrinology & Metabolism.

Ueno, A. e. (2020). *"Sarcopenia as a risk factor of severe laboratory adverse events in breast cancer patients receiving perioperative epirubicin plus cyclophosphamide therapy."*. Supportive Care in Cancer.

Urzì, A. G. (2023). *"Ketogenic Diet and Breast Cancer: Recent Findings and Therapeutic Approaches."*. Nutrients.

Uslu, C. E. (2024). *Cancer resistance and metastasis are maintained through oxidative phosphorylation.* Cancer Letters.

Vaccari, S. e. (2023). *Implant-Based Breast Reconstruction: Impact of Body Mass Index on Postoperative Complications and Aesthetic Results: A 5-Year, Single-Center Study.* Aesthetic Surgery Journal.

Van Boekel, M. A. (1993). *"Antimutagenic effects of casein and its digestion products."*. Food and chemical toxicology.

Van de Roovaart, H. J. (2024). *"Safety and efficacy of vitamin B in cancer treatments: A systematic review."*. Journal of Oncology Pharmacy Practice.

Van den Berg, M. M. (2017). *Weight change during chemotherapy in breast cancer patients: a meta-analysis.* BMC cancer.

Van der Gaag, M. S. (2001). *"Alcohol consumption stimulates early steps in reverse cholesterol transport."*. Journal of lipid research.

van Duursen, M. B. (2011). *"Genistein induces breast cancer-associated aromatase and stimulates estrogen-dependent tumor cell growth in in vitro breast cancer model."*. Toxicology.

van Enst, W. A. (2014). *"Investigation of publication bias in meta-analyses of diagnostic test accuracy: a meta-epidemiological study."*. BMC medical research methodology.

van Vliet, S. N. (2015). *"The skeletal muscle anabolic response to plant- versus animal-based protein consumption."*. The Journal of nutrition.

van Zwieten, A. e. (2024). *"Consideration of overadjustment bias in guidelines and tools for systematic reviews and meta-analyses of observational studies is long overdue."*. International Journal of Epidemiology.

Vander H., M. G. (2009). *"Understanding the Warburg effect: the metabolic requirements of cell proliferation."*. Science.

Vander, H. e. (2009). *Understanding the Warburg effect: the metabolic requirements of cell proliferation.* Science.

Vardavas, C. I. (2010). *"Cardiovascular disease risk factors and dietary habits of farmers from Crete 45 years after the first description of the Mediterranean diet."*. European Journal of Preventive Cardiology.

Veilleux, J. C. (2019). *"The relationship between distress tolerance and cigarette smoking: A systematic review and synthesis."*. Clinical psychology review.

Verbelen, H. e. (2014). *"Breast edema in breast cancer patients following breast-conserving surgery and radiotherapy: a systematic review."*. Breast cancer research and treatment.

Vernooij, R. W. (2019). *"Patterns of red and processed meat consumption and risk for cardiometabolic and cancer outcomes: a systematic review and meta-analysis of cohort studies."*. Annals of internal medicine.

Veronese, N. a.-Y. (2019). *"The effects of calorie restriction, intermittent fasting and vegetarian diets on bone health."*. Aging clinical and experimental research.

Vila, J. S. (2015). *"Overall survival according to type of surgery in young (≤ 40 years) early breast cancer patients: a systematic meta-analysis comparing breast-conserving surgery versus mastectomy."*. The Breast.

Vincent-Johnson, A. B. (2023). *"Diet and metabolism in CKD-related metabolic acidosis."*. Seminars in Nephrology.

Vin-Raviv, N. e. (2018). *"Sleep disorder diagnoses and clinical outcomes among hospitalized breast cancer patients: a nationwide inpatient sample study."*. Supportive Care in Cancer.

Violi, F. e. (2016). *"Interaction between dietary vitamin K intake and anticoagulation by vitamin K antagonists: is it really true?: a systematic review."*. Medicine.

Virtanen, J. K. (2022). *"Vitamin D supplementation and prevention of cardiovascular disease and cancer in the Finnish Vitamin D Trial: a randomized controlled trial."* . The American journal of clinical nutrition.

Vogtmann, E. e. (2013). *"Association between sleep and breast cancer incidence among postmenopausal women in the Women's Health Initiative."*. Sleep.

Waked, K. e. (2017). *"Systematic review: the oncological safety of adipose fat transfer after breast cancer surgery."*. The Breast.

Walker, A. J. (2016). *"When are breast cancer patients at highest risk of venous thromboembolism? A cohort study using English health *care data."*. Blood, The Journal of the American Society of Hematology.

Walker, J. e. (2022). *"A systematic review of pharmacologic and cell-based therapies for treatment of lymphedema (2010-2021).".* Journal of Vascular Surgery: Venous and Lymphatic Disorders.

Walker, J. e. (2023). *Chemotherapy-induced weight gain in early-stage breast cancer: a prospective matched cohort study reveals associations with inflammation and gut dysbiosis.* BMC medicine.

Wall, B. T. (2016). *"Short-term muscle disuse lowers myofibrillar protein synthesis rates and induces anabolic resistance to protein ingestion.".* American journal of physiology-endocrinology and metabolism.

Wanandi, S. I. (2017). *"Impact of extracellular alkalinization on the survival of human CD24-/CD44+ breast cancer stem cells associated with cellular metabolic shifts.".* Brazilian Journal of Medical and Biological Research.

Wanchai, A. a. (2019). *"Effects of weight-lifting or resistance exercise on breast cancer-related lymphedema: a systematic review.".* International journal of nursing sciences.

Wang, C. Z. (2015). *"Commonly used dietary supplements on coagulation function during surgery.".* Medicines.

Wang, G.-J. N. (2002). *"The role of dopamine in motivation for food in humans: implications for obesity.".* Expert opinion on therapeutic targets.

Wang, H. e. (2021). *"Impact of body mass index on pathological complete response following neoadjuvant chemotherapy in operable breast cancer: a meta-analysis.".* Breast Cancer .

Wang, H. e. (2024). *"Impact of body mass index on pathological response after neoadjuvant chemotherapy: results from the I-SPY 2 trial.".* Breast Cancer Research and Treatment.

Wang, M. J. (2021). *"Do obese breast cancer patients have more complications and a longer length of stay after mastectomy than nonobese patients?* The American Surgeon.

Wang, P. e. (2022). *"Effects of walking on fatigue in cancer patients: a systematic review and meta-analysis.".* Cancer Nursing.

Wang, P. e. (2022). *"Effects of walking on fatigue in cancer patients: a systematic review and meta-analysis."*. Cancer Nursing.

Wang, T. A. (2020). *"Deimplementation of the choosing wisely recommendations for low-value breast cancer surgery: a systematic review."*. JAMA surgery.

Wang, X. e. (2016). *"Red and processed meat consumption and mortality: dose–response meta-analysis of prospective cohort studies."*. Public health nutrition.

Wang, Z. e. (2022). *"Knowledge atlas of the involvement of glutamate and GABA in alcohol use disorder: A bibliometric and scientometric analysis."*. Frontiers in Psychiatry.

Warburg, O. (1956). *On Respiratory Impairment in Cancer Cells*. Science.

Ward, L. C. (2019). *"Bioelectrical impedance analysis for body composition assessment: reflections on accuracy, clinical utility, and standardisation."*. European journal of clinical nutrition.

Waterman, M. e. (2022). *Orthorexia symptoms and disordered eating behaviors in young women with cancer*. Eating behaviors.

Watson, N. L. (2018). *"Cigarette craving and stressful social interactions: The roles of state and trait social anxiety and smoking to cope."*. Drug and alcohol dependence.

Weaver, S. H. (2023). *"Experiences and perceptions of nurses working night shift: a qualitative systematic review."* . JBI evidence synthesis.

Weber, D. D.-G. (2018). *"Ketogenic diet in cancer therapy."*. Aging.

Wei, L. e. (2021). *"Serotonin deficiency is associated with delayed gastric emptying."*. Gastroenterology.

Wei, Y. e. (2020). *"Soy intake and breast cancer risk: A prospective study of 300,000 Chinese women and a dose–response meta-analysis."*. European journal of epidemiology.

Weikert, C. e. (2020). *"Vitamin and mineral status in a vegan diet."*. Deutsches Ärzteblatt International.

Weimann, A. e. (2021). *ESPEN practical guideline: Clinical nutrition in surgery*. Clinical Nutrition.

Weinberg, M. S. (2018). *"Beyond sarcopenia: characterization and integration of skeletal muscle quantity and radiodensity in a curable breast cancer population."*. The breast journal.

Weissman, S. e. (2020). "*The diverse involvement of cigarette smoking in pancreatic cancer development and prognosis.*". Pancreas.

Whitaker-Menezes, D. e. (2011). "*Evidence for a stromal-epithelial "lactate shuttle" in human tumors: MCT4 is a marker of oxidative stress in cancer-associated fibroblasts.*". Cell cycle.

Whitcomb, D. C. (2007). "*Human pancreatic digestive enzymes.*". Digestive diseases and sciences.

Whitfield, J. B. (2013). "*Metabolic and biochemical effects of low-to-moderate alcohol consumption.*". Alcoholism: Clinical and Experimental Research.

WHO. (2018). "*Global status report on alcohol and health 2018 [Internet]. Vol. 65, Global status report on alcohol. 2018. 74–85 p.*". Global status report on alcohol. 2018. 74–85 p.

WHO. (2018). "*Noncommunicable diseases country profiles 2018.*".

WHO. (2020). "*Smoking and COVID-19: Scientific brief.*".

Wijma, B. A. (2016). "*Silence, shame and abuse in health care: theoretical development on basis of an intervention project among staff.*". BMC medical education.

Wilcox, C. E. (2021). "*The food addiction concept: History, controversy, potential pitfalls, and promises.*". Food Addiction, Obesity, and Disorders of Overeating: An Evidence-Based Assessment and Clinical Guide.

Wilder R, W. M. (1922). "*The threshold of ketogenesis.*". Journal of Biological Chemistry.

Wilder, R. (1921). "*The effects of ketonemia on the course of epilepsy.*". Mayo Clin Proc. Vol. 2.

Willett, W. C. (1995). "*Mediterranean diet pyramid: a cultural model for healthy eating.*". The American journal of clinical nutrition.

Williams, D. E. (2021). "*Indoles derived from glucobrassicin: Cancer chemoprevention by indole-3-carbinol and 3, 3'-diindolylmethane.*". Frontiers in Nutrition.

Witard, O. C. (2021). "*Making sense of muscle protein synthesis: a focus on muscle growth during resistance training.*". International journal of sport nutrition and exercise metabolism.

Witkiewicz, A. K. (2012). *Using the "reverse Warburg effect" to identify high-risk breast cancer patients: stromal MCT4 predicts poor clinical outcome in triple-negative breast cancers*. Cell cycle.

Wolfe, R. R. (2006). *"The underappreciated role of muscle in health and disease."*. The American journal of clinical nutrition.

Wong, G. e. (2020). *"The impact of smoking on adjuvant breast cancer radiation treatment: A systematic review."*. Cancer Treatment and Research Communications.

Wong, J. e. (2012). *"Short-term preoperative smoking cessation and postoperative complications: a systematic review and meta-analysis."*. Canadian Journal of Anesthesia.

Woo, H. D. (2012). *"Differential influence of dietary soy intake on the risk of breast cancer recurrence related to HER2 status."*. Nutrition and cancer.

Woodall, M. J. (2020). *"The effects of obesity on anti-cancer immunity and cancer immunotherapy."*. Cancers.

Woodward, M. a.-P. (1992). *"Biochemical evidence of persistent heavy smoking after a coronary diagnosis despite self-reported reduction: analysis from the Scottish Heart Health Study."*. European heart journal.

Wopat, H. e. (2023). *"Body composition and chemotherapy toxicity among women treated for breast cancer: a systematic review."*. Journal of Cancer Survivorship.

Worbe, Y. e. (2014). *"Serotonin depletion induces 'waiting impulsivity' on the human four-choice serial reaction time task: cross-species translational significance."*. Neuropsychopharmacology.

Wu, L. e. (2022). *"Smoking cessation, weight gain, and risk for type 2 diabetes: a prospective study."*. International Journal of Public Health.

Wu, P. S. (2018). *"Waist-to-hip ratio is a better predictor than body mass index for morbidity in abdominally based breast reconstruction."*. Microsurgery.

Wu, Q. a. (2023). *"Autophagy and breast cancer: connected in growth, progression, and therapy."*. Cells.

Wu, W. K. (2012). *"The autophagic paradox in cancer therapy."*. Oncogene.

Wu, Y. W.-W. (2020). *"Total red meat, unprocessed red meat, processed meat and risk of breast cancer-a pooled analysis of 23 cohort studies."*. Cancer Research.

Xia, J. e. (2017). *"Cigarette smoking and chronic kidney disease in the general population: a systematic review and meta-analysis of prospective cohort studies."*. Nephrology Dialysis Transplantation.

Xiao, Y. e. (2022). *The prognosis of bladder cancer is affected by fatty acid metabolism, inflammation, and hypoxia.* Frontiers in Oncology.

Xie, Y. e. (2021). *"Risk factors related to acute radiation dermatitis in breast cancer patients after radiotherapy: a systematic review and meta-analysis."*. Frontiers in oncology.

Xie, Y. e. (2021). *Risk factors related to acute radiation dermatitis in breast cancer patients after radiotherapy: a systematic review and meta-analysis.* Frontiers in oncology.

Xu, S. e. (2021). *Hair chemicals may increase breast cancer risk: a meta-analysis of 210319 subjects from 14 studies.* PLoS one.

Yücel, K. B. (2024). *"Visceral obesity and sarcopenia as predictors of efficacy and hematological toxicity in patients with metastatic breast cancer treated with CDK 4/6 inhibitors."*. Cancer Chemotherapy and Pharmacology.

Yabe, S. e. (2021). *"Association between skin flap necrosis and sarcopenia in patients who underwent total mastectomy."*. Asian Journal of Surgery.

Yakın, E. P. (2022). *"Distinguishing between healthy and pathological orthorexia: a cluster analytic study."*. Eating and Weight Disorders-Studies on Anorexia, Bulimia and Obesity.

Yalçın, N. e. (2019). *"Drug-induced nutritional disorders."*. Clinical Science of Nutrition.

Yang, J. e. (2012). *"Effect of dietary fiber on constipation: a meta analysis."*. World journal of gastroenterology.

Yang, J. e. (2023). *"Short sleep duration and the risk of nonalcoholic fatty liver disease/metabolic associated fatty liver disease: a systematic review and meta-analysis."*. Sleep and Breathing.

Yang, Z.-J. e. (2022). *"Effects and mechanisms of curcumin for the prevention and management of cancers: An updated review."*. Antioxidants.

Ye, F. e. (2015). *"Efficacy of and patient compliance with a ketogenic diet in adults with intractable epilepsy: a meta-analysis."*. Journal of clinical neurology (Seoul, Korea).

Yeomans, M. R. (2004). *"Palatability: response to nutritional need or need-free stimulation of appetite?."*. British Journal of Nutrition.

Yezhelyev, M. e. (2013). *"Complications of latissimus dorsi flap breast reconstruction in overweight and obese patients."*. Annals of plastic surgery.

Young, K. L. (2023). *"Influence of alcohol consumption and alcohol metabolism variants on breast cancer risk among Black women: results from the AMBER consortium."*. Breast Cancer Research.

Young, K. L. (2023). *"Influence of alcohol consumption and alcohol metabolism variants on breast cancer risk among Black women: results from the AMBER consortium."*. Breast Cancer Research.

Yustisia, I. S. (2017). *"Effects of extracellular modulation through hypoxia on the glucose metabolism of human breast cancer stem cells."*. Journal of Physics: Conference.

Zöllner, J. P. (2015). *"Changes of pH and energy state in subacute human ischemia assessed by multinuclear magnetic resonance spectroscopy."*. Stroke.

Zagami, P. e. (2024). *"Cardiotoxicity of agents used in patients with breast cancer."*. JCO Oncology Practice.

Zagouri, F. e. (2015). *"Discrepancies between ESMO and NCCN breast cancer guidelines: An appraisal."*. The Breast.

Zaki, A. e. (2008). *"Interventions in the preoperative clinic for long term smoking cessation: a quantitative systematic review."*. Database of Abstracts of Reviews of Effects (DARE): Quality-assessed Reviews .

Zang, J. e. (2015). *"The association between dairy intake and breast cancer in Western and Asian populations: a systematic review and meta-analysis."*. Journal of breast cancer.

Zaromskyte, G. e. (2021). *"Evaluating the leucine trigger hypothesis to explain the post-prandial regulation of muscle protein synthesis in *young and older adults: a systematic review."*. Frontiers in Nutrition.

Zeraatkar, D. e. (2019). *"Effect of lower versus higher red meat intake on cardiometabolic and cancer outcomes: a systematic review of randomized trials."*. Annals of internal medicine.

Zeraatkar, D. e. (2019). *"Red and processed meat consumption and risk for all-cause mortality and cardiometabolic outcomes: a systematic review and meta-analysis of cohort studies."*. Annals of internal medicine.

Zewenghiel, L. H. (2018). *"Impact of body mass index on the efficacy of endocrine therapy in patients with metastatic breast cancer-A retrospective two-center cohort study."*. The Breast.

Zhang, S.-L. e. (2016). *"Effect of vitamin B supplementation on cancer incidence, death due to cancer, and total mortality: A PRISMA-compliant cumulative meta-analysis of randomized controlled trials."*. Medicine.

Zhang, S.-L. e. (2016). *"Effect of vitamin B supplementation on cancer incidence, death due to cancer, and total mortality: A PRISMA-compliant cumulative meta-analysis of randomized controlled trials."*. Medicine.

Zhang, X.-M. e. (2020). *"Sarcopenia as a predictor of mortality in women with breast cancer: a meta-analysis and systematic review."*. BMC cancer.

Zhang, Y. e. (2014). *"Impact of preoperative anemia on relapse and survival in breast cancer patients."*. BMC cancer.

Zhao, J. e. (2023). *"Association between daily alcohol intake and risk of all-cause mortality: a systematic review and meta-analyses."*. JAMA network open.

Zhao, Q. e. (2020). *"The impact of COPD and smoking history on the severity of COVID-19: A systemic review and meta-analysis."*. Journal of medical virology.

Zhao, T.-T. e. (2019). *"Dietary isoflavones or isoflavone-rich food intake and breast cancer risk: A meta-analysis of prospective cohort studies."*. Clinical nutrition.

Zhao, Z. e. (2017). *"Association between consumption of red and processed meat and pancreatic cancer risk: a systematic review and meta-analysis.".* Clinical Gastroenterology and Hepatology.

Zhao, Z. Z. (2017). *"Red and processed meat consumption and gastric cancer risk: A systematic review and meta-analysis.".* Oncotarget.

Zheng, Y. e. (2024). *"Effect of physical exercise on the emotional and cognitive levels of patients with substance use disorder: a meta-analysis.".* Frontiers in Psychology.

Zickgraf, H. F. (2021). *"Orthorexia nervosa vs. healthy orthorexia: relationships with disordered eating, eating behavior, and healthy lifestyle choices.".* Eating and Weight Disorders-Studies on Anorexia, Bulimia and Obesity.

Ziouziou, I. e. (2021). *"Association of processed meats and alcohol consumption with renal cell carcinoma: a worldwide population-based study.".* Nutrition and Cancer.

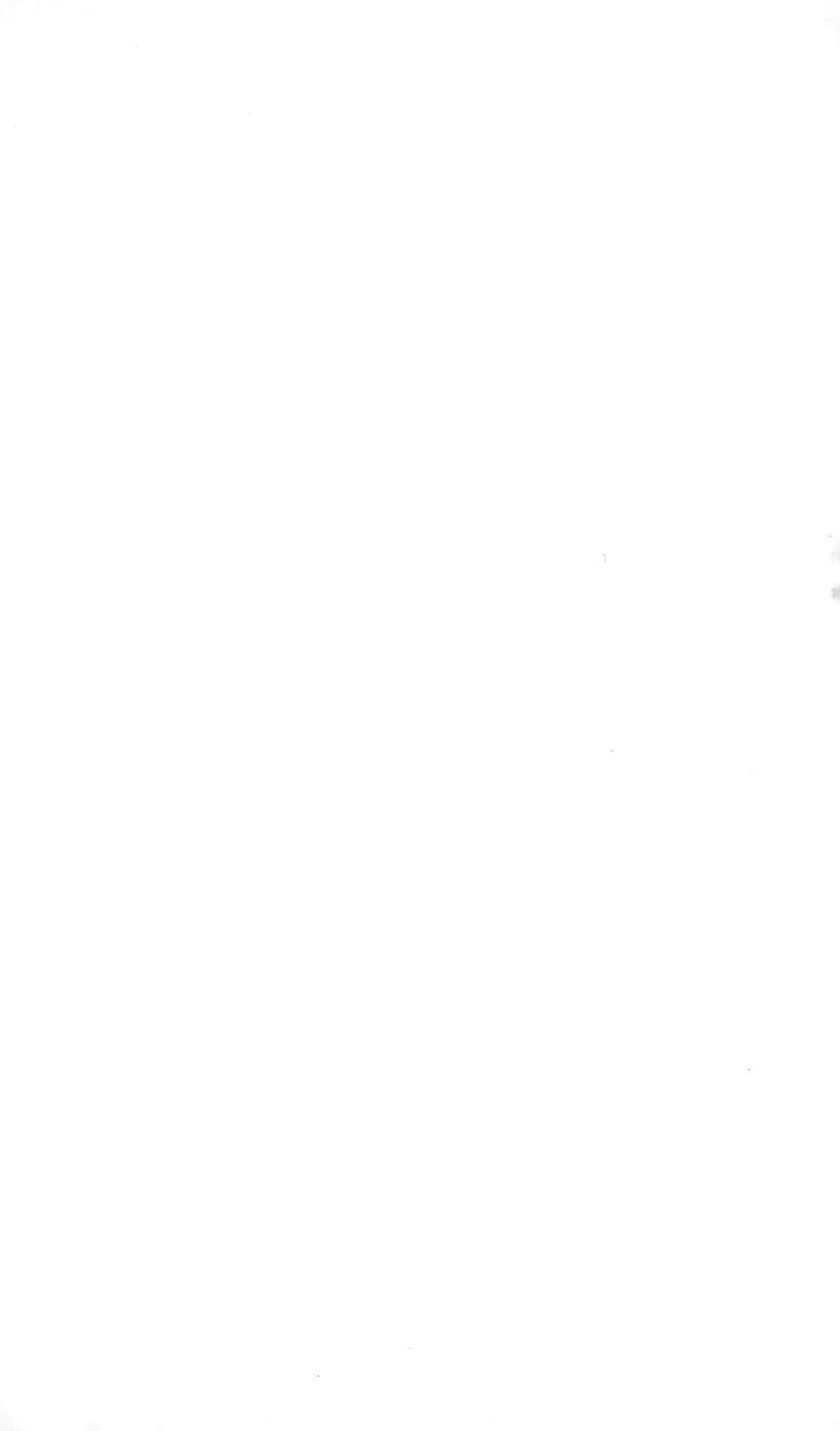

Made in the USA
Columbia, SC
06 September 2024

ddb64cbb-410d-40df-83ad-ee8c87db218bR01